Treatment for Hoarding Disorder

T0177786

EDITOR-IN-CHIEF

David H. Barlow, PhD

SCIENTIFIC
ADVISORY BOARD

Anne Marie Albano, PhD

Gillian Butler, PhD

David M. Clark, PhD

Edna B. Foa, PhD

Paul J. Frick, PhD

Jack M. Gorman, MD

Kirk Heilbrun, PhD

Robert J. McMahon, PhD

Peter E. Nathan, PhD

Christine Maguth Nezu, PhD

Matthew K. Nock, PhD

Paul Salkovskis, PhD

Bonnie Spring, PhD

Gail Steketee, PhD

John R. Weisz, PhD

G. Terence Wilson, PhD

✓Treatments *That Work*™

Treatment for Hoarding Disorder

Workbook

Second Edition

Gail Steketee • Randy O. Frost

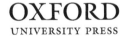

OXFORD

UNIVERSITY PRESS

OXFORD
UNIVERSITY PRESS

Oxford University Press is a department of the University of Oxford.
It furthers the University's objective of excellence in research, scholarship,
and education by publishing worldwide.

Oxford   New York
Auckland   Cape Town   Dar es Salaam   Hong Kong   Karachi
Kuala Lumpur   Madrid   Melbourne   Mexico City   Nairobi
New Delhi   Shanghai   Taipei   Toronto

With offices in
Argentina   Austria   Brazil   Chile   Czech Republic   France   Greece
Guatemala   Hungary   Italy   Japan   Poland   Portugal   Singapore
South Korea   Switzerland   Thailand   Turkey   Ukraine   Vietnam

Oxford is a registered trademark of Oxford University Press in the UK
and certain other countries.

Published in the United States of America
by Oxford University Press
198 Madison Avenue, New York, NY 10016

© Oxford University Press 2014

All rights reserved. No part of this publication may be reproduced, stored in
a retrieval system, or transmitted, in any form or by any means, without the prior
permission in writing of Oxford University Press, or as expressly permitted by law,
by license, or under terms agreed with the appropriate reproduction rights organization.
Inquiries concerning reproduction outside the scope of the above should be sent to the
Rights Department, Oxford University Press, at the address above.

You must not circulate this work in any other form
and you must impose this same condition on any acquirer.

ISBN 978–0–19–933494–0

About Treatments *ThatWork*™

One of the most difficult problems confronting patients with various disorders and diseases is finding the best help available. Everyone is aware of friends or family who have sought treatment from a seemingly reputable practitioner, only to find out later from another doctor that the original diagnosis was wrong or the treatments recommended were inappropriate or perhaps even harmful. Most patients, or family members, address this problem by reading everything they can about their symptoms, seeking out information on the Internet or aggressively "asking around" to tap knowledge from friends and acquaintances. Governments and health care policymakers are also aware that people in need do not always get the best treatments—something they refer to as *variability in health care practices*.

Now health care systems around the world are attempting to correct this variability by introducing *evidence-based practice*. This simply means that it is in everyone's interest that patients get the most up-to-date and effective care for a particular problem. Health care policymakers have also recognized that it is very useful to give consumers of health care as much information as possible, so that they can make intelligent decisions in a collaborative effort to improve physical health and mental health. This series, Treatments *That Work*™, is designed to accomplish just that. Only the latest and most effective interventions for particular problems are described in user-friendly language. To be included in this series, each treatment program must pass the highest standards of evidence available, as determined by a scientific advisory board. Thus, when individuals suffering from these problems or their family members seek out an expert clinician who is familiar with these interventions and decides that they are appropriate, patients will have confidence they are receiving the best care available. Of course, only your health care professional can decide on the right mix of treatments for you.

This particular program presents the latest version of a cognitive–behavioral treatment for excessive hoarding and acquiring behavior. Formerly thought to be a type of obsessive–compulsive disorder, hoarding disorder is now recognized as its own, distinct problem and this updated version of the treatment program reflects the newest research on how to best treat it. Hoarding disorder can have devastating consequences, not only on individuals suffering from this problem, but also their families and, in many cases, their neighbors and public health authorities, who may be called in when excessive debris and garbage accumulates outside the house. The essence of this problem is the inability to throw away unneeded items and the urge to acquire unnecessary, excessive possessions. In many cases, houses become so cluttered that it becomes impossible to use the living space in any reasonable kind of way. This problem is estimated to afflict approximately 1% to 2% of the population, and this treatment program was the first effective, evidence-based treatment created to help those with the disorder. Now, after several years of new research and refined development, Drs. Steketee and Frost have updated the program and incorporated the latest findings and techniques to help those who hoard and acquire. In an evaluation of this treatment, individuals reduced clutter in their homes by approximately 50% after just several months of treatment and continued to make substantial progress. These results make this program a beacon of hope for those who have suffered its consequences, sometimes for decades. Although this program must be carried out under the guidance of a skilled clinician who has been trained in its use, it offers the best prospect yet of relief from the considerable suffering associated with hoarding.

David H. Barlow, Editor-in-Chief,
Treatments *ThatWork*™
Boston, MA

Contents

Acknowledgments

The authors gratefully acknowledge the contributions to this book from all of the participants in our research studies—especially those in our treatment trials, which form the basis for this therapy for hoarding disorder. We also acknowledge our clinical and research colleagues from around the world whose fine work has enabled us to advance our understanding of hoarding disorder. We could not have done this work without our own longstanding collaboration and partnership as researchers and co-authors. Oxford University Press has been highly supportive throughout the writing process, with help from Sarah Harrington, Andrea Zekus, and Prasad Tangudu and others who have facilitated the planning, writing, and editing of this Guide and Workbook. Gail is especially blessed to have the support of her husband Brian McCorkle throughout the many months of writing and editing for the revised Guide and Workbook. Randy has special thanks for his wife Sue, whose support and encouragement have helped make this work possible.

Treatment for Hoarding Disorder

Chapter 1

Introduction

Goals

- To understand compulsive hoarding
- To learn about this treatment program and what it will involve

What Is Hoarding?

Personal possessions play a large role in everyone's life. The things we own provide us with comfort, convenience, and pleasure. They can help us to live full and happy lives. But sometimes, when we lose control over them, they can cause wrack and ruin. Recognition of this fact has been slow in coming. The first systematic study of hoarding did not occur until the early 1990s. Since then, however, a great deal of research has taught us much about hoarding. In 2013, the American Psychiatric Association made hoarding a distinct disorder in its diagnostic code, the *Diagnostic and Statistical Manual of Mental Disorders* (5th ed.; DSM-5). The primary symptom of hoarding is the saving of so many possessions that they interfere with the ability to live. Specifically, the accumulation of objects clutters the living spaces of the home so they can't be used for their intended purposes. This leads to significant problems in social, personal, occupational, and financial functioning and can cause considerable emotional distress. In addition, acquiring problems are evident in most cases and include acquiring free items, picking up things others have thrown away, and compulsive buying. Excessive acquiring and saving both lead to clutter in the home that interferes with the ability to use rooms comfortably. To qualify as a true hoarding problem, it is the living areas of the home that must be cluttered. Having attics, closets, and basements full of stuff does not rise to the level of a disorder.

We know that hoarding typically begins in childhood and often runs in families. In fact, recent research has indicated a genetic component to this problem. Hoarding is typically chronic and doesn't get better without treatment. Hoarding problems are remarkably common, affecting somewhere between 2% and 6% of the population. The consequences of hoarding can be devastating, including death from fire or being crushed by toppling stacks of objects. It can have a destructive effect on families as well. You can learn more about the phenomena of hoarding in our book *Stuff: Compulsive Hoarding and the Meaning of Things* (2010, Houghton Mifflin Harcourt).

In addition to possible genetic vulnerability, people with Hoarding Disorder (HD) appear to process information differently and to think about possessions differently. Because of these problems, people learn to acquire and save too many things, and to avoid decision-making, discarding, and organizing. How that happens is outlined briefly below.

Information Processing Problems

Many people who suffer from HD have attention-deficit problems that make it difficult for them to sustain attention, especially to a difficult task. These attention deficit and hyperactivity disorder (ADHD)-type problems lead to inefficient and ineffective attempts to clear clutter. You may have noticed that when you sit down to begin clearing clutter, your attention gets drawn away to other things. Before long you find yourself looking through a magazine rather than making decisions about what to keep and what to get rid of.

Efficient organization of possessions requires the ability to combine similar objects into meaningful categories for filing and/or storage. People with a hoarding problem have difficulty in this regard. They seem to see each possession as complex, unique, and irreplaceable. Before discarding, each feature of the object must be considered and the possibility of finding something this unusual again must be estimated. Attempts at organization/discarding often involve examining an object only to place it back in the pile of things from which it was drawn. The result is a pile of unrelated objects, both important and unimportant, that get "churned" during attempts to organize and result in "losing" important things.

Difficulties with confidence in memory may complicate the processing of information for people who hoard. They often lack confidence in their ability to remember things, and many also believe that it is important to remember almost everything. To avoid the possibility of forgetting information from something they read, they keep the paper or magazine instead. In addition, they want to keep important things in sight as reminders of their existence. To them, putting anything out of sight means they may not remember they have it. The sight of an object appears to increase its value such that seemingly unimportant things (for example, scraps of paper with unrecognized phone numbers) are elevated to the same status as important things (for example, paychecks). Because those who hoard define so many things as important, nearly everything must be left in sight. At the time a possession is being used, it has a high level of "importance" and consequently gets put on top of the pile—in sight. Subsequent items take over as "important" and go on top of the previous "important" item, eventually burying it in the pile. The pile consists of layers of once "important" possessions.

People who hoard often have a strong visual attraction to objects. They want to keep possessions in sight, so they end up in the middle of the room. At the same time, they notice individual objects but seem to fail to see the whole. Quite a number of people with HD have what we call "clutter blindness." They fail to notice the extent of clutter in their own home.

Another related part of the information processing picture is a kind of overly complex thinking. People with HD appear to generate more ideas and thoughts about possessions than do other people (that is, thoughts about uses, value, aesthetics, opportunities, etc.). These details about possessions are so complex and plentiful that distinguishing important from unimportant details becomes very difficult. This makes it hard to make decisions about whether to keep or get rid of possessions, and about where and how to store them.

Evaluating costs and benefits of saving is another complication. When trying to discard or organize, thoughts about the cost of discarding dominate the person's thinking. Little or no consideration is given to the cost of saving a possession or the benefit of getting rid of it. The same problem is evident for resisting urges to acquire.

Two aspects of thinking play a role in the problem of hoarding. The first of these is thinking styles and the second is specific beliefs about possessions. One is a *way* of thinking and the other is the *content* of that thinking. Regarding thinking styles, for a long time psychologists and psychiatrists have recognized that certain patterns of thinking influence how we feel about ourselves and the world. For example, Dr. David Burns (1989) identified a series of common errors in reasoning that lead to emotional distress. Characteristic thinking patterns common in compulsive hoarding include:

1. *All-or-nothing thinking*: Black-and-white thinking exemplified by extreme words like "most," "everything," and "nothing," often accompanying perfectionistic standards. An example is "It seems like *everything* in this box is just so important."

2. *Overgeneralization*: Generalization from a single event to all situations, using words like "always" or "never." Examples are "I will *never* find this if I move it" and "If I don't keep this, I'll *always* regret it."

3. *Jumping to conclusions*: Predicting negative outcomes without supporting facts, akin to catastrophizing (see below). An example is "You know I'll need this just as soon as I decide to get rid of it."

4. *Catastrophizing*: Exaggerating the severity of possible outcomes—for example, "If I throw it away, I'll go crazy thinking about it."

5. *Discounting the positive*: Positive experiences are not counted, as in the statement: "Yes, I've created a filing system, but that isn't really progress because there is so much more to do."

6. *Emotional reasoning*: Emotions are used instead of logic so feelings substitute for facts. For example, "If I feel uncomfortable about throwing this away, it means I should keep it."

7. *Moral reasoning*: "Should" statements (including "must," "ought," and "have to") accompanied by guilt and frustration

often driven by perfectionistic standards: "I have to keep this health information in case something happens to John."

8. *Labeling*: Attaching a negative label to oneself or others, such as "I can't find my electric bill. I'm such an idiot" and "She's just greedy and wants all my stuff."

9. *Under- and overestimating*: Underestimating the time to accomplish a task or one's ability to cope or, conversely, overestimating one's ability to complete a task or the emotional costs of doing so. For example, "I'll be able to read all those newspapers eventually."

The content of thoughts about possessions is what gives objects meaning. People with hoarding problems find meaning in possessions to a far greater extent than most people. Interestingly, people without hoarding problems find the same sorts of meaning in their possessions, but the intensity, range, and volume is not as great. Possessions can have a wide range of meanings, including the ones described below. You will recognize some of them in yourself.

Common Meanings of Possessions

Beauty	Finding beauty and aesthetic appeal in unusual objects
Memory	Belief/fear that memories will be lost without objects or that objects contain or preserve memories
Utility/opportunity/uniqueness	Seeing the usefulness of virtually anything. seeing opportunities presented by objects that others don't
Sentimental	Attaching emotional significance to objects; anthropomorphism
Comfort/safety	Perceiving objects (and related behaviors like shopping) as providing emotional comfort; objects as sources of safety (safety signals)
Identity/validation of self-worth	Belief that objects are part of the person or represent who the person can become; objects as representation of self-worth; getting rid of possessions feels like losing a part of oneself
Control	Concern that others will control one's possessions or behavior
Mistakes	Perfectionistic concern about making mistakes or about the condition or use of possessions
Responsibility/waste	Strong beliefs about not wasting possessions, about polluting the environment, or about using possessions responsibly
Socializing	Buying or collecting items provides social contact not available in other ways

When the meanings we give to our possessions become intense, they can provide us with a positive feeling at the sight of them. The aesthetic qualities of a simple vase can provide intense pleasure. A cookbook that generates images of cooking dinner for friends can fulfill one's sense of identity as a social host and/or a good chef. Imagining an otherwise disposable item being put to good use rather than thrown into the landfill makes people feel good. Thinking of an inanimate object as having feelings can provide a sense of companionship. In each of these cases, the positive feelings are short-lived, yet they can be very intense. Similarly, the feelings associated with acquiring a new object can be exhilarating, at least initially. These kinds of experiences make acquiring and saving objects more likely. In this way, the meanings that we give to our possessions reinforce our behaviors of acquiring and saving them. But the reinforcement is short-lived. The possessions often go onto a pile somewhere and are seldom seen or used again. Now they have become part of the problem rather than a source of real pleasure.

Just as powerful as the short-term positive reinforcement we receive from acquiring and saving possessions is the sense of discomfort associated with the thought of getting rid of them. The meanings we give to possessions help create this discomfort and make us avoid the distress we feel at the thought of losing them. For instance, a belief about the importance of retaining information from a newspaper might create discomfort at the thought of recycling it: "I might lose an important opportunity." That discomfort can be avoided entirely by just keeping the paper. If a cookbook provides an image of what life could be like, the thought of getting rid of it feels like losing that dream. Simply saving the cookbook and returning it to the pile makes that sad feeling go away. People with hoarding problems frequently report that when they see something they would like to acquire, the thought of NOT acquiring it fills them with a sense of loss, and they imagine that this opportunity will never come to them again. The easiest way to escape these uncomfortable feelings is to acquire the item. Thus, the simple act of setting something down on top of a pile avoids the whole uncomfortable process of making decisions about possessions.

The intervention program described here grew out of our work with many clients whom we studied intensively in individual and group treatment. The therapy consisted of weekly office visits to work on reducing acquiring, learning skills for organizing, sorting possessions, making decisions about what to get rid of, changing beliefs, and reducing avoidance of difficult emotions and tasks. Regular but less frequent home sessions enabled people to gain skills in their own home environment so successful outcomes could be sustained when the therapy ended.

Over the past few years, this therapy has been used with many clients who exhibited moderate to severe hoarding problems and often had other problems like attention-deficit disorder, depression, marital problems, social anxiety, and health problems. Some of these clients functioned very well on their jobs and in their social lives but were unable to make headway with severe clutter that filled all living spaces and rendered the home useless for all but bathing and sleeping. Others had significant problems in their work, social, and family lives, but they improved nonetheless.

We have completed a waitlist-controlled study in which we randomly assigned clients with HD to either immediate treatment or to a 12-week waitlist followed by the treatment (Steketee, Frost, Tolin, Rasmussen, & Brown, 2010). Treatment consisted of 26 sessions over 9 to 10 months, with home visits occurring every month. Of the 43 people who began the therapy program, only 6 (14%) did not continue for various reasons, such as deciding to work on another problem they considered more important or inability to find the time to devote to the treatment. These clients ranged in age from 42 to 66 and about 35% were men. Even after only 12 weeks, clients who received the therapy showed significantly more reduction in their hoarding symptoms (27%) compared to those on the waitlist (11%). Although it may not seem like it, statistically, this difference is considered very large. After 26 sessions, the patients who completed treatment experienced a 39% reduction in their hoarding symptoms, an even larger effect. In addition, over 80% of the clients who completed the treatment rated themselves as "much" or "very much" improved. These findings are very positive, especially for a problem that has not responded well to medications or to other psychotherapy methods. In fact, at this time there are no standard medications that have consistently been shown to improve hoarding, nor is there any other form of psychotherapy that we know of that is effective for hoarding.

Brief Description of the Program

Throughout this treatment program you will learn various skills and techniques for dealing with your hoarding and excessive acquiring. In the first few therapy sessions, your clinician will help you assess your hoarding problem and how it affects your life. He or she will want to visit you in your home to get a better idea of the extent of your hoarding problem. Together, you will also construct a model to help explain your hoarding behavior based on the meanings you have for your possessions. Your model will help you to better understand your symptoms and how they developed. Later therapy sessions focus on preparing for treatment and selecting the most effective intervention methods for your specific case. In every session your clinician will work with you to keep you motivated.

The treatment will teach you problem-solving and decision-making skills. You'll develop a personal organizing plan and put it into effect in your own home. You will be asked to participate in sorting and decision-making exercises, which will gradually help you get used to the discomfort of making hard choices, getting rid of items, and not acquiring things if this is a problem for you. With your clinician's help, you will sort through your possessions one by one and room by room and learn to discard, recycle, and donate the things you decide not to keep. This work will include examining how you think about your possessions and the meanings you have assigned to them that might or might not be true. You'll be asked to take different perspectives on your acquiring and saving preferences to help you change thinking that contributes to the clutter problem. Finally, you will learn strategies for anticipating and coping with stressors and maintaining your new habits. All of this work will be done collaboratively with your clinician, who will ask you to observe closely your own thoughts, emotions, and behaviors and will invite your views on the best ways to make the changes you need.

You will probably struggle with motivation to keep working on hoarding when you find yourself feeling anxious, guilty, or down. Old habits, even ones you know are bad, are hard to break. This treatment program is designed to help you do just that in a supportive relationship with your clinician, who will help you stay focused on the tasks ahead.

Using This *Workbook*

This *Workbook* contains all the forms, worksheets, and exercises you need to participate in this treatment. You will move through this book under the direction of your clinician. Each chapter includes a list of goals and is focused on helping you learn specific methods or techniques to assess your problem, understand it, and modify your thoughts, feelings, and behaviors. Interactive forms and worksheets are included in each chapter where they are first introduced. Additional copies are included in the Appendix and can also be downloaded from the Treatments *ThatWork*™ website at www.oup.com/us/ttw. Follow your clinician's instructions for using these forms. Homework exercises are listed at the end of each chapter, and you and your clinician will agree on what you can do each week to practice new skills, thinking, and behaviors.

This *Workbook* is an important component of your treatment, and you will refer to it regularly. You should bring it to every session and talk to your clinician about the best place to keep it so you can avoid misplacing or losing it in the clutter of your home.

References

Burns, D. (1989). *Feeling good handbook*. New York: Morrow.

Steketee, G., Frost, R. O., Tolin, D. F., Rasmussen, J., & Brown, T. A. (2010). Waitlist controlled trial of cognitive behavior therapy for hoarding disorder. *Depression and Anxiety*, *27*, 476–484.

Chapter 2

Assessing Hoarding Problems

Goals

- To complete a Personal Session Form

- To complete assessment measures

- To allow your clinician to visit you in your home

- To choose a family member or friend or other person as your "coach"

Self-Assessment

The Personal Session Form on the next page is yours to complete each time you meet with your clinician, whether in the office or in your home or in another setting you and your clinician arrange. The Appendix of this *Workbook* contains extra Personal Session Forms for your use throughout the treatment. Use these forms to make notes about your agenda, points you want to recall from the session, homework assignments, and any topics you want to discuss next time. Take care to complete the form with enough detail to be able to remember what you learned from the session. At the end of the treatment, you and your clinician will review your forms to pick out the methods that worked best for you, so be sure that you write enough down that you can recall the details when the time comes to refer back to your notes.

Use the tests included on the next few pages to determine whether or not you have a problem with hoarding and to what degree it affects your life. Brief instructions for scoring are provided in the Appendix. Your clinician will work with you to score these measures and discuss the results with you.

Personal Session Form

Initials: _____   Session #: _____   Date: _____

Agenda:

_____

_____

_____

Main Points:

_____

_____

_____

_____

_____

_____

Homework:

_____

_____

_____

_____

_____

_____

To Discuss Next Time:

_____

_____

_____

_____

_____

More Personal Session Forms are available in the Appendix at the back of this *Workbook*.

Hoarding Rating Scale (HRS)

Date: _____

1. Because of the clutter or number of possessions, how difficult is it for you to use the rooms in your home?

0 ---------- 1 ----------- 2 ------------ 3 ------------ 4 ------------ 5 ------------ 6------------ 7 ------------ 8

| Not at all Difficult | Mild | Moderate | Severe | Extremely Difficult |

2. To what extent do you have difficulty discarding (or recycling, selling, giving away) ordinary things that other people would get rid of?

0 ------------ 1 ------------ 2 ------------ 3 ------------ 4 ------------ 5 ------------ 6 ---------- 7 ----------- 8

| Not at all Difficult | Mild | Moderate | Severe | Extremely Difficult |

3. To what extent do you currently have a problem with collecting free things or buying more things than you need or can use or can afford? [Use the scale below]

0 ------------- 1 ------------- 2 ------------ 3 ------------ 4 ------------ 5 ------------ 6 ------------ 7 ------------- 8

| No problem | | | | Extreme |

    0 = no problem
    2 = mild problem, occasionally (less than weekly) acquires items not needed,
        or acquires a few unneeded items
    4 = moderate, regularly (once or twice weekly) acquires items not needed, or
        acquires some unneeded items
    6 = severe, frequently (several times per week) acquires items not needed,
        or acquires many unneeded items
    8 = extreme, very often (daily) acquires items not needed, or acquires large
        numbers of unneeded items

4. To what extent do you experience emotional distress because of clutter, difficulty discarding or problems with buying or acquiring things?

0 ------------- 1 ------------- 2 ------------- 3 ----------- 4 ------------- 5 ----------- 6 ------------- 7 ----------- 8

| None/ Not at all | Mild | Moderate | Severe | Extremely |

5. To what extent do you experience impairment in your life (daily routine, job / school, social activities, family activities, financial difficulties) because of clutter, difficulty discarding, or problems with buying or acquiring things?

0 ------------- 1 ----------- 2 ------------- 3 ----------- 4 ------------- 5 ------------- 6 ----------- 7 ------------ 8

| None/ Not at all | Mild | Moderate | Severe | Extremely |

Table 2.1 Cutoff Scores and Typical Hoarding Rating Scale (HRS) Scores in Hoarding and Non-Hoarding Samples (Tolin, Frost, & Steketee, 2010)

	Cutoff scores (scores at or above this indicate hoarding)	Average scores for people with HD (standard deviation)	Average scores for people without HD (standard deviation)
Total HRS	14	24.22 (5.7)	3.34 (5.0)
#1 Clutter	3	5.18 (1.4)	0.64 (1.1)
#2 Difficulty Discarding	4	5.10 (1.4)	0.82 (1.4)
#3 Acquisition	2	4.08 (1.9)	0.75 (1.3)
#4 Distress	3	4.83 (1.3)	0.73 (10)
#5 Interference	3	5.03 (1.4)	0.42 (1.0)

Saving Inventory – Revised

For each question below, circle the number that corresponds most closely to your experience DURING THE PAST WEEK.

0 -------------- 1 ------------------ 2 ---------------- 3 --------------- 4

None	A little	A moderate amount	Most/Much	Almost All/ Complete

	None	A little	A moderate amount	Most/Much	Almost All/Complete
1. How much of the living area in your home is cluttered with possessions? (Consider the amount of clutter in your kitchen, living room, dining room, hallways, bedrooms, bathrooms, or other rooms).	0	1	2	3	4
2. How much control do you have over your urges to acquire possessions?	0	1	2	3	4
3. How much of your home does clutter prevent you from using?	0	1	2	3	4
4. How much control do you have over your urges to save possessions?	0	1	2	3	4
5. How much of your home is difficult to walk through because of clutter?	0	1	2	3	4

For each question below, circle the number that corresponds most closely to your experience DURING THE PAST WEEK.

0 --------------------- 1 ------------------- 2 ------------------ 3 ------------------- 4

	Not at all	Mild	Moderate	Considerable/ Severe	Extreme
6. To what extent do you have difficulty throwing things away?	0	1	2	3	4
7. How distressing do you find the task of throwing things away?	0	1	2	3	4
8. To what extent do you have so many things that your room(s) are cluttered?	0	1	2	3	4
9. How distressed or uncomfortable would you feel if you could not acquire something you wanted?	0	1	2	3	4
10. How much does clutter in your home interfere with your social, work or everyday functioning? Think about things that you don't do because of clutter.	0	1	2	3	4
11. How strong is your urge to buy or acquire free things for which you have no immediate use?	0	1	2	3	4

Saving Inventory – Revised *continued*

For each question below, circle the number that corresponds most closely to your experience DURING THE PAST WEEK:

0	1	2	3	4
Not at all	Mild	Moderate	Considerable/ Severe	Extreme

12. To what extent does clutter in your home cause you distress?	0	1	2	3	4
13. How strong is your urge to save something you know you may never use?	0	1	2	3	4
14. How upset or distressed do you feel about your acquiring habits?	0	1	2	3	4
15. To what extent do you feel unable to control the clutter in your home?	0	1	2	3	4
16. To what extent has your saving or compulsive buying resulted in financial difficulties for you?	0	1	2	3	4

For each question below, circle the number that corresponds most closely to your experience DURING THE PAST WEEK.

0	1	2	3	4
Never	Rarely	Sometimes/ Occasionally	Frequently/ Often	Very Often

17. How often do you avoid trying to discard possessions because it is too stressful or time consuming?	0	1	2	3	4
18. How often do you feel compelled to acquire something you see? e.g., when shopping or offered free things?	0	1	2	3	4
19. How often do you decide to keep things you do not need and have little space for?	0	1	2	3	4
20. How frequently does clutter in your home prevent you from inviting people to visit?	0	1	2	3	4
21. How often do you actually buy (or acquire for free) things for which you have no immediate use or need?	0	1	2	3	4
22. To what extent does the clutter in your home prevent you from using parts of your home for their intended purpose? For example, cooking, using furniture, washing dishes, cleaning, etc.	0	1	2	3	4
23. How often are you unable to discard a possession you would like to get rid of?	0	1	2	3	4

Table 2.2 Cutoff Scores and Typical Saving Inventory–Revised (SI-R) Scores in Hoarding and Non-Hoarding Samples (Frost, Steketee, & Grisham, 2004)

	Cutoff scores (scores at or above this indicate hoarding)	Average scores for people with HD (standard deviation)	Average scores for people without HD (standard deviation)
Total SI-R	41	62.0 (12.7)	23.7 (13.2)
Clutter	17	26.9 (6.6)	8.2 (7.1)
Difficulty Discarding	14	19.8 (5.0)	9.2 (5.0)
Excessive Acquisition	9	15.2 (5.4)	6.4 (3.6)

Clutter Image Rating

Date: _____

Using the 3 series of pictures (CIR: Living Room, CIR: Kitchen, and CIR: Bedroom), please select the picture that best represents the amount of clutter for each of the rooms of your home. Put the number on the line below.

Please pick the picture that is closest to being accurate, even if it is not exactly right.

If your home does not have one of the rooms listed, just put NA for "not applicable" on that line.

Room	Number of closest corresponding picture (1–9)
Living Room	_____
Kitchen	_____
Bedroom #1	_____
Bedroom #2	_____

Also, please rate other rooms in your house that are affected by clutter on the lines below. Use the *CIR: Living Room* pictures to make these ratings.

Dining room	_____	
Hallway	_____	
Garage	_____	
Basement	_____	
Attic	_____	
Car	_____	
Other	_____	Please specify: _____

Scores above 3 in any room are cause for concern.

Clutter Image Rating: Living Room

Please select the photo below that most accurately reflects the amount of clutter in your room.

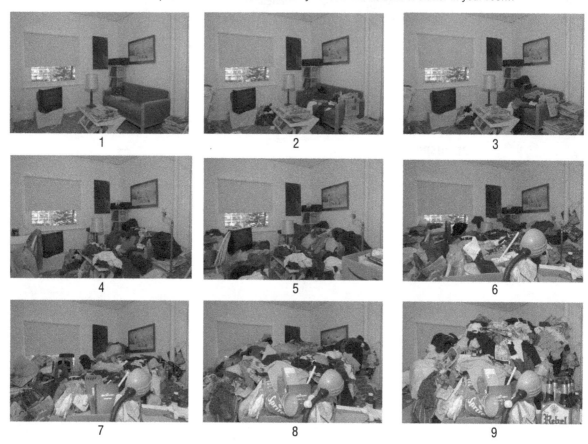

Figure 2.1

Clutter Image Rating Scale: Living Room

Clutter Image Rating Scale: Kitchen

Please select the photo below that most accurately reflects the amount of clutter in your room.

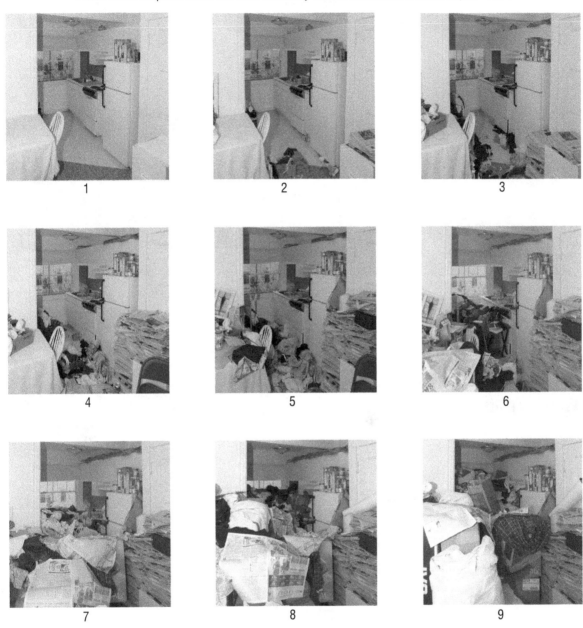

Figure 2.2

Clutter Image Rating Scale: Kitchen

Clutter Image Rating: Bedroom

Please select the photo that most accurately reflects the amount of clutter in your room.

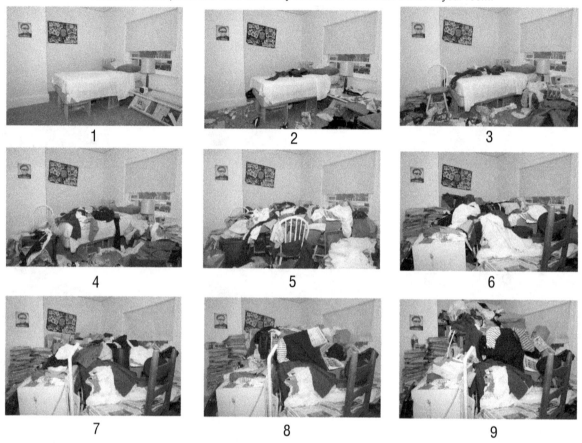

1 2 3

4 5 6

7 8 9

Figure 2.3

Clutter Image Rating Scale: Bedroom

Table 2.3 Typical Clutter Image Rating Scores (CIR) in Hoarding and Non-Hoarding Samples (Tolin, Frost, Steketee, & Renaud, 2008)

	Average scores for people with HD (standard deviation)	Average scores for people without HD (standard deviation)
Living Room	3.7 (2.0)	1.3 (1.0)
Kitchen	3.4 (1.6)	1.2 (0.6)
Bedroom	4.1 (1.6)	1.3 (0.8)

Saving Cognitions Inventory

Date: _____

Use the following scale to indicate the extent to which you had each thought when you were deciding whether to throw something away DURING THE PAST WEEK. (If you did not try to discard anything in the past week, indicate how you would have felt if you had tried to discard.)

```
1 -------------- 2 -------------- 3 -------------- 4 -------------- 5 -------------- 6 -------------- 7
   not at all                        sometimes                          very much
```

1. I could not tolerate it if I were to get rid of this.	1 2 3 4 5 6 7
2. Throwing this away means wasting a valuable opportunity.	1 2 3 4 5 6 7
3. Throwing away this possession is like throwing away a part of me.	1 2 3 4 5 6 7
4. Saving this means I don't have to rely on my memory.	1 2 3 4 5 6 7
5. It upsets me when someone throws something of mine away without my permission.	1 2 3 4 5 6 7
6. Losing this possession is like losing a friend.	1 2 3 4 5 6 7
7. If someone touches or uses this, I will lose it or lose track of it.	1 2 3 4 5 6 7
8. Throwing some things away would feel like abandoning a loved one.	1 2 3 4 5 6 7
9. Throwing this away means losing a part of my life.	1 2 3 4 5 6 7
10. I see my belongings as extensions of myself; they are part of who I am.	1 2 3 4 5 6 7
11. I am responsible for the well-being of this possession.	1 2 3 4 5 6 7
12. If this possession may be of use to someone else, I am responsible for saving it for them.	1 2 3 4 5 6 7
13. This possession is equivalent to the feelings I associate with it.	1 2 3 4 5 6 7
14. My memory is so bad I must leave this in sight or I'll forget about it.	1 2 3 4 5 6 7
15. I am responsible for finding a use for this possession.	1 2 3 4 5 6 7
16. Throwing some things away would feel like part of me is dying.	1 2 3 4 5 6 7
17. If I put this into a filing system, I'll forget about it completely.	1 2 3 4 5 6 7
18 I like to maintain sole control over my things.	1 2 3 4 5 6 7
19. I'm ashamed when I don't have something like this when I need it.	1 2 3 4 5 6 7
20. I must remember something about this, and I can't if I throw this away.	1 2 3 4 5 6 7
21. If I discard this without extracting all the important information from it, I will lose something.	1 2 3 4 5 6 7
22. This possession provides me with emotional comfort.	1 2 3 4 5 6 7
23. I love some of my belongings the way I love some people.	1 2 3 4 5 6 7
24. No one has the right to touch my possessions.	1 2 3 4 5 6 7

Table 2.4 Typical Saving Cognitions Inventory (SCI) Scores in Hoarding and Non-Hoarding Samples (Steketee, Frost, & Kyrios, 2003)

	Average scores for people with HD (standard deviation)	Average scores for people without HD (standard deviation)
Total SCI	95.9 (31.0)	42.2 (20.9)
Emotional Attachment	37.7 (16.0)	14.8 (8.7)
Control	15.8 (4.2)	8.4 (5.1)
Responsibility	22.3 (8.2)	10.4 (6.0)
Memory	20.3 (8.1)	8.8 (4.8)

Activities of Daily Living for Hoarding (ADL-H)

Date: _____

Sometimes clutter in the home can prevent you from doing ordinary activities. For each of the following activities, please circle the number that best represents the degree of difficulty you experience in doing this activity because of the clutter or hoarding problem. If you have difficulty with the activity for other reasons (for example, unable to bend or move quickly due to physical problems), do not include this in your rating. Instead, rate only how much difficulty you would have **due to hoarding**. If the activity is not relevant to your situation (for example, you don't have laundry facilities or animals), circle Not Applicable (NA).

Activities affected by clutter or hoarding problem	Can do it easily	Can do it with a little difficulty	Can do it with moderate difficulty	Can do it with great difficulty	Unable to do	Not Applicable
1. Prepare food	1	2	3	4	5	NA
2. Use refrigerator	1	2	3	4	5	NA
3. Use stove	1	2	3	4	5	NA
4. Use kitchen sink	1	2	3	4	5	NA
5. Eat at table	1	2	3	4	5	NA
6. Move around inside the house	1	2	3	4	5	NA
7. Exit home quickly	1	2	3	4	5	NA
8. Use toilet	1	2	3	4	5	NA
9. Use bath/shower	1	2	3	4	5	NA
10. Use bathroom sink	1	2	3	4	5	NA
11. Answer door quickly	1	2	3	4	5	NA
12. Sit in sofa/chair	1	2	3	4	5	NA
13. Sleep in bed	1	2	3	4	5	NA
14. Do laundry	1	2	3	4	5	NA
15. Find important things (such as bills, tax forms, etc.)	1	2	3	4	5	NA

Table 2.5 Typical Activities of Daily Living for Hoarding (ADL-H) Scores in Hoarding and Non-Hoarding Samples (Frost, Hristova, Steketee, & Tolin, 2013)

	Average scores for people with HD	Average scores for people without HD Controls
Total ADL-H	2.20 (.74)	1.15 (.75)

We recommend classifying the scores as:

1.0–1.4	None to minimal
1.5–2.0	Mild
2.1–3.0	Moderate
3.1–4.0	Severe
4.1–5.0	Extreme

Safety Questions

Date: _____

Sometimes the clutter in your home can cause safety problems. Please circle the number below that best indicates how much of a problem you have with the following conditions in your home:

Safety problems in the home	None	A little	Somewhat/ moderate	Substantial	Severe
1. Is there structural damage to the floors, walls, roof, or other parts of your home?	1	2	3	4	5
2. Is your water not working?	1	2	3	4	5
3. Is your heat not working?	1	2	3	4	5
4. Does any part of your house pose a fire hazard? (stove covered with paper, flammable objects near the furnace, etc.)	1	2	3	4	5
5. Would medical emergency personnel have difficulty moving equipment through your home?	1	2	3	4	5
6. Are exits from your home blocked?	1	2	3	4	5
7. Is it unsafe to move up or down the stairs or along other walkways?	1	2	3	4	5

A score of 2 or above on any question is meaningful and needs attention.

Home Environment Index

Date: _____

Clutter and hoarding problems can sometimes lead to sanitation problems. Please circle the answer that best fits the current situation in the home.

To what extent are the following situations present in the home?

1. Fire hazard
    0 = No fire hazard
    1 = Some risk of fire (for example, lots of flammable material)
    2 = Moderate risk of fire (for example, flammable materials near heat source)
    3 = High of fire (for example, flammable materials near heat source; electrical hazards, etc.)

2. Moldy or rotten food
    0 = None
    1 = A few pieces of moldy or rotten food in kitchen
    2 = Some moldy or rotten food throughout kitchen
    3 = Large quantity of moldy or rotten food in kitchen and elsewhere

3. Dirty or clogged sink
    0 = Sink empty and clean
    1 = A few dirty dishes with water in sink
    2 = Sink full of water, possibly clogged
    3 = Sink clogged with evidence that it has overflowed onto counters, etc.

4. Standing water (in sink, tub, other container, basement, etc.)
    0 = No standing water
    1 = Some water in sink/tub
    2 = Water in several places, especially if dirty
    3 = Water in numerous places, especially if dirty

5. Human/animal waste/vomit
    0 = No human waste, animal waste, or vomit visible
    1 = No human waste or vomit; no animal waste or vomit outside cage or box
    2 = Some animal or human waste or vomit visible (for example, in unflushed toilet)
    3 = Animal or human waste or vomit on floors or other surfaces

6. Mildew or mold
    0 = No mildew or mold detectable
    1 = Small amount of mildew or mold in limited amounts and expected places (for example, on edge of shower curtain or refrigerator seal)
    2 = Considerable, noticeable mildew or mold
    3 = Widespread mildew or mold on most surfaces

7. Dirty food containers
    0 = All dishes washed and put away
    1 = A few unwashed dishes
    2 = Many unwashed dishes
    3 = Almost all dishes are unwashed

8. Dirty surfaces (floors, walls, furniture, etc.)
   0 = Surfaces completely clean
   1 = A few spills, some dirt or grime
   2 = More than a few spills, may be a thin covering of dirt or grime in living areas
   3 = No surface is clean; dirt or grime covers everything

9. Piles of dirty or contaminated objects (bathroom tissue, hair, toilet paper, sanitary products, etc.)
   0 = No dirty or contaminated objects on floors, surfaces, etc.
   1 = Some dirty or contaminated objects present around trash cans or toilets
   2 = Many dirty or contaminated objects fill bathroom or area around trash cans
   3 = Dirty or contaminated objects cover the floors and surfaces in most rooms

10. Insects
    0 = No insects are visible
    1 = A few insects visible; cobwebs and/or insect droppings present
    2 = Many insects and droppings are visible; cobwebs in corners
    3 = Swarms of insects; high volume of droppings; many cobwebs on household items

11. Dirty clothes
    0 = Dirty clothes placed in hamper; none are lying around
    1 = Hamper is full; a few dirty clothes lying around
    2 = Hamper is overflowing; many dirty clothes lying around
    3 = Clothes cover the floor and many other surfaces (bed, chairs, etc.)

12. Dirty bed sheets/linens
    0 = Bed coverings very clean
    1 = Bed coverings relatively clean
    2 = Bed coverings dirty and in need of washing
    3 = Bed coverings very dirty and soiled

13. Odor of house
    0 = No odor
    1 = Slight odor
    2 = Moderate odor; may be strong in some parts of house
    3 = Strong odor throughout house

During the last month, how often did you (or someone in your home) do each of the following activities?

14. Do the dishes
    0 = Daily or every 2 days; 15 to 30 times per month
    1 = 1-2 times a week; 4 to 10 times per month
    3 = Every other week; 2 to 3 times per month
    3 = Rarely; 0 times per month

15. Clean the bathroom
    0 = Daily or every 2 days; more than 10 times per month
    1 = 1-2 times a week; 4 to 10 times per month
    2 = Every other week; 2 to 3 times per month
    3 = Never; 0 times per month

A score of 2 or above on any question warrants attention.
Rasmussen, Steketee, Frost, & Tolin (in press).

Home Visit

At some point within the first few sessions of your treatment, your clinician will want to visit you in your home. During this first visit, your clinician will walk around with you to understand the amount and types of items you have saved and where the clutter has accumulated. Both of you will discuss how to begin work on sorting, organizing, and removing clutter.

In addition, assemble a box or bag of typical saved items for use during your clinic appointments to learn and practice new skills. This box should contain random clutter from your home, such as junk mail, newspapers, magazines, small objects, receipts, notes, ticket stubs, clothing, shoes, books, etc. These clutter items should be selected mainly from the room in which treatment will begin.

If you are living with someone who is affected by your hoarding problem, your clinician may want to meet with you and him or her during the home visit as well.

Picking a Coach

Some family members or friends who are calm, thoughtful, and empathic people can be enlisted as coaches during the intervention. Discuss this with your clinician to determine whether anyone qualifies for this role. The role of your "coach" is to help you engage in various assignments throughout the course of your treatment. Instructions for Coaches are provided in the Appendix at the back of this *Workbook* to help guide the person with whom you plan to work.

Homework

- Review the material about hoarding from chapter 1.

- Complete self-assessment questionnaires.

- Assemble a box or bag of items to bring to office appointments for sorting.

References

Frost, R.O., Hristova, V., Steketee, G., & Tolin, D.F. (2013). Activities of daily living in hoarding disorder (ADL-H). *Journal of Obsessive Compulsive and Related Disorders, 2,* 85–90.

Frost, R.O., Steketee, G., & Grisham, J. (2004). Measurement of compulsive hoarding: Saving Inventory-Revised. *Behaviour Research and Therapy, 42,* 1163–1182.

Frost, R.O., Steketee, G., Tolin, D.F., & Renaud, S. (2008). Development and validation of the Clutter Image Rating. *Journal of Personality and Behavioral Assessment. 30,* 193–203.

Rasmussen, J., Steketee, G., Frost, R.O., Tolin, D.F., & Brown, T.A. (in press). Assessing squalor in hoarding: The Home Environment Index. *Community Mental Health Journal.*

Steketee, G., Frost, R.O., & Kyrios, M. (2003). Cognitive aspects of compulsive hoarding. *Cognitive Therapy and Research, 27,* 463–479..

Tolin, D.F., Frost, R.O., & Steketee, G. (2010). A brief interview for assessing compulsive hoarding: The Hoarding Rating Scale. *Psychiatry Research, 30,* 147–152.

Chapter 3

Developing Your Personal Hoarding Model

Goals

- To develop a personal model of your hoarding problem

Look back at the Personal Session Form from the last session to remind yourself of what happened in your last session, your homework assignment, and what topics you want to discuss at the next session.

Building Your Hoarding Model

You probably have many questions about why this has happened to you and why you think about possessions differently from other people. Gaining control over your hoarding problem depends upon your understanding of why you acquire and keep so many items. Your clinician will help you develop a model of your hoarding problem based on what we know about the disorder. Now that you've read the "What Is Hoarding" section of chapter 1, you have a general idea about hoarding. In this chapter we will help you construct a model of what drives your hoarding behavior. This will give you the knowledge to overcome it.

As you recall from chapter 1, many factors contribute to your hoarding, including personal and family vulnerabilities, information processing problems, the meanings your possessions hold for you, and avoidance behaviors. Your clinician will help you fill in the boxes in the model pictured below. An additional blank Hoarding Model is included in the appendices.

Personal and Family Vulnerabilities

We know that hoarding behavior runs in families and may be partly genetic. Include in your model a note about any of your immediate relatives who have hoarding tendencies. Other vulnerabilities to include are your own problems with depression, social anxiety, or other psychological problems. Also note any traumas you may have experienced that you think contribute to your hoarding (e.g., assault, abuse, etc.). List any physical constraints you have (e.g., back or joint problems, breathing problems, etc.). Finally, include early life experiences that may have contributed to your hoarding. For instance, indicate if your parents were especially concerned about wasting resources or were overly sentimental with respect to possessions.

Information Processing Problems

As you may recall from chapter 1, there are several information processing problems that are common in hoarding, including attention problems, categorization/organization, memory, perception, complex thinking, and decision-making difficulties. List any of these that apply to you in your model. Discuss these with your therapist to determine how they will affect the treatment.

Meaning of Possessions

The meanings possessions have for you are the driving force behind your saving and acquiring. They include thoughts you have about the importance of possessions, as well as emotional attachments to them.

Recall the list of meanings that are attached to possessions from chapter 1: beauty, memory, utility/opportunity/uniqueness, sentimental, comfort/safety, identity/self-worth, control, mistakes, responsibility/waste, socializing. Each one of these types of meanings is associated with thoughts people have about possessions. Below we have listed some examples of thoughts associated with each of these meanings that we have collected from our clients. Many of them are similar to the items on the Saving Cognitions Inventory you completed in chapter 2. Look though them and pick out the ones that you recognize in yourself. Then include those in the model in Figure 3.1.

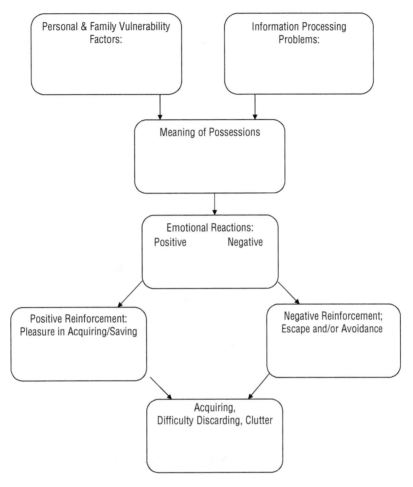

Figure 3.1

Hoarding Model for _____ (Client's Initials)

Beauty

This is too pretty to throw away.

I must keep everything that is purple.

It is a shame to lose something so beautiful.

Memory

Saving things means I don't have to rely on my memory.

If I put things into a filing system, I'll forget about them.

In my life, the past has been very important to me so I try to hold onto it.

I must keep things in sight, or I'll forget about them.

If I throw this away, I'll lose the memories associated with it.

Utility/Opportunity/Uniqueness

Getting rid of this means losing a valuable opportunity.

I'll never find another one like it.

I just might need this some day.

Getting rid of this will mean losing information that might be important.

If an object has any potential value, I must save it.

This is so unique that there is nothing else like it in the world.

If I can imagine a use for something, then it must be worth saving.

If I think I might need something, it's more likely that I will really need it.

If I don't keep/get this information now, I won't be able to get it again.

Sentimental

Throwing this away is like throwing away a part of me.

Losing this is like losing a friend.

Throwing this away feels like abandoning a loved one.

Comfort/Safety

Without this, I'll feel vulnerable.

I can't tolerate getting rid of this.

I feel most comfortable around my stuff.

My stuff is like a cocoon that makes me feel better.

Identity/Self-Worth

This possession represents who I am.

If I throw too much away, there will be nothing left of me.

If I imagine life without my stuff, it feels empty.

Getting rid of my cookbooks feels like giving up on my dream of
being a cook.

Control

If someone touches my things, I'll lose them or I'll lose track of them.

People who use my things will wreck them.

I don't want anyone touching my stuff.

I could only give this to a worthy person who would appreciate it
properly.

Before I get rid of something, I have to know that it's going to a
good home.

Mistakes

I have to read and understand every article before I can discard the
newspaper.

I must organize everything exactly right.

Throwing something out and finding I needed it later would
be awful.

If I can't do it right, there is no sense in doing it at all.

Responsibility/Waste

I'm responsible for not wasting this.

Throwing something away might be wasting a valuable
opportunity.

I am responsible for finding a use for these things.

I am responsible for the well-being of my possessions.

If I have something that someone else might want, I should save it
for them.

Socializing

My stuff keeps me connected with the world and other people.

If I don't go to the garage/tag sales on Saturdays, I won't see my friends anymore.

Emotional Reactions

In your model in Figure 3.1, list the emotional reactions you have to the kinds of meanings you have identified. Here are some examples provided by our former clients:

Joy—from finding a long-lost object

Elation—from acquiring a new object

Sadness—from finding a broken toy at the bottom of the pile

Guilt—from throwing away something that I should have kept instead

Anger—at someone from mishandling my possessions

Loss—feeling like I've lost a part of my life by throwing something away

Frustration—from how difficult it is to make decisions about my stuff

Lonely—from being trapped by the clutter

Brief Thought Record

The Brief Thought Record shown may be helpful when working with your clinician to develop your model of hoarding. Use the blank form to record triggering events, thoughts, and beliefs, as well as the emotions and behaviors that follow. Additional copies are provided in the Appendix so you can complete them as homework.

Brief Thought Record

Initials: _____   Date: _____

Trigger Situation	Thought or Belief	Emotions	Actions/Behaviors

Model of Acquiring

To help with including information about acquiring in your model, it is useful to keep track of acquiring behaviors over a period of time. Models for acquiring have more positive feelings and fewer negative ones than models for cluttering or difficulty discarding. Start with the Acquiring Form below to help you become aware of every item you bring home in a week's time. Tracking this is often illuminating and will help you and your therapist develop a model for understanding the factors that drive your acquiring actions.

Acquiring Form

Make a list of the types of items you typically bring into your home and how you acquired them. Think about items you acquired in the past week and record what items you acquire during the coming week. Do not include groceries or other perishable goods. Rate how uncomfortable you would feel if you didn't acquire this item when you saw it.

Item and where you typically find it	Discomfort if not acquired (0 to 100)

To understand how your hoarding developed and is maintained, it is useful to do a very detailed analysis of what happens in real time while you make decisions about acquiring or saving. We call this a "functional analysis" because we try to see how the feelings, thoughts, and behaviors function together—that is, how one thing leads to the other. To do this requires information about your personal experience (your thoughts, feelings, and behaviors) on a moment-to-moment basis. It is easiest to see this by selecting an episode in the last day or two in which you made a decision about acquiring or about saving. If your clinician went through this with you during your last session, try it on your own by picking a very recent event and filling in the boxes in Figure 3.2 for an acquiring event or Figure 3.3 for a situation in which you considered getting rid of something but decided to save it. Each event will be different, so you may not use all the boxes or you may need more boxes.

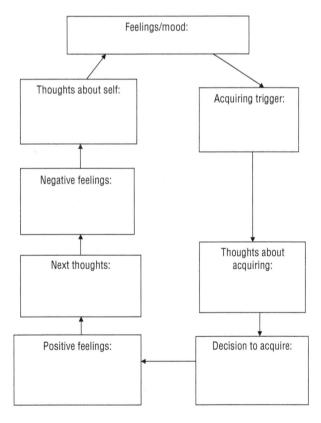

Figure 3.2
Functional Analysis of Acquiring Episode

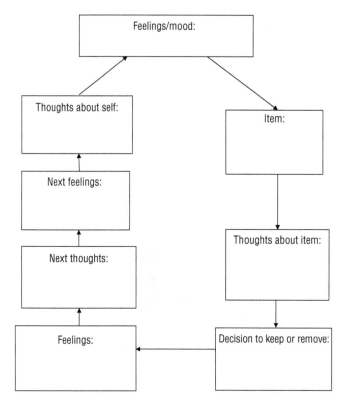

Figure 3.3

Functional Analysis of Discarding Episode

Homework

- Work on the model (Fig. 3.1) at home to identify any additional components that contribute to hoarding or acquiring.

- Monitor thoughts and feelings using the Brief Thought Record form while sorting at home or when acquiring.

- Complete the Acquiring Form to obtain a full list of the types of items accumulated in recent weeks and months.

- Work on a functional analysis (Fig. 3.2) after an incident of acquiring to capture the sequence of triggering events, thoughts, feelings and actions.

- Work on a functional analysis (Fig. 3.3) after an effort to discard an item to capture the sequence of triggering events, thoughts, feelings and actions.

Chapter 4

Planning Your Treatment

Goals

- To establish treatment goals and set rules for treatment

- To complete the visualization exercises

  Remember to use the Personal Session Form to make notes about your agenda, points you want to recall from the session, homework assignments, and any topics you want to discuss with your clinician during the next session. Copies of the form are included in the Appendix.

Treatment Goals and Rules

At this point you will work with your clinician to establish your treatment goals and the rules you'll follow during therapy. If you have chosen someone to be your "coach," as discussed in the previous chapter, he or she should be present during this planning phase.

The Goals Form below lists goals for treatment that our clients typically identify and includes a section titled "Personal Goals." Here you will identify your own goals for the coming weeks and months.

The following list of rules will ensure that your treatment progresses in a manner and at a pace you can manage. Your clinician will discuss these in further detail during the treatment planning session. You and your clinician may decide on other rules you would like to add.

Goals

Treatment Goals

1. Understand why I hoard.

2. Create living space I can use.

3. Get organized to find things more easily and make them more accessible.

4. Improve my decision-making.

5. Reduce my compulsive buying or acquiring.

6. Reduce clutter.

Personal Goals

My main goals in this treatment are:

1. _____

2. _____

3. _____

4. _____

5. _____

6. _____

7. _____

8. _____

9. _____

10. _____

Treatment Rules

1. The clinician may not touch or remove any item without explicit permission.

2. The client makes all decisions about possessions.

3. Treatment proceeds systematically—by room, type of item, or difficulty of the task.

4. The client and clinician will establish an organizing plan before sorting possessions.

5. The client will think aloud while sorting possessions to understand and evaluate thoughts and beliefs better.

6. Only handle it once (OHIO)—or at most twice.

7. Treatment will proceed in a flexible manner.

Visualization Exercises

To understand your motivation for entering treatment for hoarding, you will complete several visualization and practice exercises. These exercises will help your clinician to plan your treatment and will also help you to clarify your thoughts and feelings about organizing, reducing clutter, and limiting acquiring.

The first exercise is to complete the Clutter Visualization Form below. For this task you will visualize the current cluttered state of a specific room in your home and record your level of discomfort as you form the image in your mind. Ideally, you will choose an important room such as the kitchen, dining room, living room, or bedroom.

The second exercise is to complete the Unclutter Visualization Form below. This time you will visualize the same room you did during the previous exercise, but without any clutter. Imagine that everything you want to keep is still there, but organized, sorted, and put in its proper place. How does this make you feel? Record your level of discomfort.

The third exercise is to complete the Acquiring Visualization Form below. For this, visualize a situation that provokes a strong urge to acquire something and record your thoughts and feelings. Then imagine leaving without the item and describe your reactions.

Clutter Visualization Form

Room: _____

A. Visualize this room with all of its present clutter. Imagine standing in the middle of the room slowly turning to see all of the clutter.

B. How uncomfortable did you feel while imagining this room with all the clutter? Use a scale from 0 to 100, where 0 = no discomfort and 100 = the most discomfort you have ever felt.

Initial Discomfort Rating: _____

C. What feelings were you having while visualizing this room?

    1. _____

    _____

    _____

    2. _____

    _____

    _____

    3. _____

    _____

    _____

D. What thoughts (beliefs, attitudes) were you having while visualizing this room?

    1. _____

    _____

    _____

    2. _____

    _____

    _____

    3. _____

    _____

    _____

Unclutter Visualization Form

Room: _____

A. Visualize this room with the clutter gone. Imagine cleared surfaces and floors, tabletops without piles, and uncluttered floors with only rugs and furniture. Don't think about where the things have gone; just imagine the room without clutter.

B. How uncomfortable did you feel while imagining this room without all the clutter? Use a scale from 0 to 100, where 0 = no discomfort and 100 = the most discomfort you have ever felt.

Initial Discomfort Rating: _____

C. What thoughts and feelings you were having while visualizing this room?

 1. _____

 _____

 2. _____

 _____

 3. _____

 _____

D. Imagine what you can do in this room now that it is not cluttered. Picture how pleasant this room will feel when you have arranged it the way you want it. Describe your thoughts and feelings.

 1. _____

 _____

 2. _____

 _____

 3. _____

 _____

E. How uncomfortable did you feel while imagining the room this way? (0 = no discomfort and 100 = the most discomfort you have ever felt)

Final Discomfort Rating: _____

Acquiring Visualization Form

Visualize a typical situation in which you have a strong urge to acquire something. In your image, don't actually pick up the item, just look at it. Please describe the location and item you imagined.

Rate how strong was your urge to acquire the item (0 = no urge to acquire, 100 = irresistible urge).

Acquiring urge: _____

What thoughts did you have while you imagined this scene?

1. _____

_____

2. _____

_____

3. _____

_____

Visualize this scene again, but this time, imagine leaving without the item. How much discomfort did you experience while imagining (0 to 100)?

Discomfort Rating _____

Please list any thoughts you think would help you to not acquire an object.

1. _____

_____

2. _____

_____

3. _____

_____

Now rate how uncomfortable you feel about leaving without the item(s) from 0 to 100.

Discomfort Rating _____

Practice Form

A. What was the item (to remove or not to acquire)? _____

_____

Initial discomfort (0 = no discomfort to 100 = maximal discomfort) _____

_____

_____

B. What did you do (not acquire, trash, recycle, give away, other)? _____

_____

_____

Discomfort rating (0 to 100)   after 10 min _____

after 20 min _____

after 30 min _____

after 40 min _____

after 50 min _____

after 1 hour _____

the next day _____

_____

C. Conclusion regarding experiment: _____

_____

_____

_____

_____

Additional copies of the Practice Form can be found in the Appendix.

Practice Exercises

During treatment your clinician will ask you to complete various homework assignments. One of these assignments is to perform practice exercises during which you get rid of (discard, recycle) a possession that may make you feel uncomfortable. After you have removed the item, you will record how you feel for the next few hours and days using the Practice Form above. Additional copies of the form are included in the Appendix.

Homework

- Think about your personal goals and record them in the "Personal Goals" section of the Goals Form.

- Monitor your thoughts and feelings during sorting, discarding, and acquiring by completing the various visualization exercises included in this chapter at home.

- Focus on your thinking while getting rid of something using the Practice Form.

Chapter 5 · *Reducing Acquiring*

Goals

- To develop questions for acquiring

- To develop an exposure hierarchy to practice reducing acquiring

- To identify and engage in pleasurable, alternative non-acquiring activities

- To learn techniques to change beliefs and use them during practice in not acquiring

Remember to use the Personal Session Form to make notes about your agenda, points you want to recall from the session, homework assignments, and any topics you want to discuss next time. Copies of the form are included in the Appendix.

Excessive Acquiring

Most individuals who suffer from hoarding problems also have difficulty with excessive acquiring, either because they are compulsive buyers or because they can't say no when offered things for free. Your clinician will help you review your Acquiring Form and your model of acquiring behaviors to help you understand how your behavior is triggered and reinforced. You and your clinician will work in a stepwise fashion to build your resistance to urges to acquire and to develop alternative pleasurable activities.

Avoiding Triggers for Acquiring

Sometimes you can control excessive acquisition by simply avoiding the triggers for acquiring episodes. For example, you can avoid going out on Saturday morning so you won't see ongoing tag/ garage sales. This strategy may work in the short term, but avoidance of acquiring cues is not likely to work over the longer term. You can't avoid acquiring cues forever, and you will find that you must avoid an ever-growing number of places. The activities in this part of your treatment will help you learn to control urges in the presence of triggers for acquiring. This will require practice in acquiring situations.

Work with your clinician to decide how to avoid situations in which you have strong urges to acquire that you are not yet prepared to manage. For example, if you have trouble resisting yard sale items, you can decide to plan other events for Saturdays when these usually happen until you are ready to face this situation. If you can't resist special sales, you might decide not to look at the newspaper ads for a few weeks to help you avoid the problem until you are prepared to handle it using the strategies in this chapter.

Focus of Attention

One thing that frequently happens during acquiring episodes is that the focus of attention becomes so narrow that people acquire without thinking clearly. They seem to forget that they did not plan to acquire and they don't have available space, money, or time to use the item. They also frequently forget that they may already have more than one of the items they are acquiring. A very simple yet effective strategy for dealing with this problem is to construct a list of questions you think you should ask yourself before acquiring something. You can then carry this list with you. When you are faced with whether or not to acquire something, just pull out your questions and answer them. If your answers indicate that it is okay to get the item, then go ahead. This method keeps the information you need to make a reasonable decision ready at hand. Some of the questions our clients have come up with in the past are listed below on the Acquiring Questions Form. Feel free to add your own questions to this list. Then make a copy that you can carry with you.

Acquiring Questions Form

- Does it fit with my own personal values?

- Do I have a real need for this item (not just a wish to have it)?

- Do I already own something similar?

- Am I only buying this because I feel bad (angry, depressed, etc.) now?

- In a week, will I regret getting this?

- Could I manage without it?

- If it needs fixing, do I have enough time to do this or is my time better spent on other activities?

- Will I actually use this item in the near future?

- Do I have a specific place to put this?

- Is this truly valuable or useful or does it just seem so because I'm looking at it now?

- Is it good quality (accurate, reliable, attractive)?

- Will *not* getting this help me solve my hoarding problem?

- _____

- _____

- _____

- _____

- _____

- _____

- _____

Additional copies of the Acquiring Questions Form can be found in the Appendix.

Establish Rules for Acquiring

If you and your clinician determine that you need to acquire fewer things, it will be helpful for you to establish rules to accomplish this goal. Work with your clinician to generate rules that help you decide when to refrain from acquiring. For example, you may decide not to acquire unless you plan to use the item in the next month, or if you have an uncluttered place in your home to put the item. Record your rules on the My Rules for Acquiring Form below.

My Rules for Acquiring Form

1. _____

2. _____

3. _____

4. _____

5. _____

Advantages and Disadvantages

One way to change beliefs about acquiring is to consider the advantages and disadvantages of acquiring something. People who acquire too many items often think about the immediate benefits of getting a new thing and forget about the costs of doing this. Use the Advantages/Disadvantages Worksheet for Acquiring below to help you think more clearly about whether you truly want to acquire an item. This worksheet has only two sections to help you think about the advantages and disadvantages of acquiring something you don't yet own. Your clinician can help you decide when to use this worksheet.

Practice Exercises for Non-acquiring

You can change your ability to tolerate your urges to acquire in much the same way you set up a physical fitness routine. You need to start by exposing yourself to places where you experience a mild urge to acquire,

Advantages/Disadvantages Worksheet for Acquiring

Specify the item(s) under consideration: _____

Advantages (Benefits) of Acquiring	Disadvantages (Costs) of Acquiring

but one that you can resist. Then you must move up to a situation that evokes a stronger urge. Your clinician will help you develop a hierarchy of increasingly difficult situations in which you would normally acquire more items than you need. For example, driving by and standing outside shops may be relatively easy for you to accomplish alone or with others, but actually going into shops without purchasing anything is likely to be harder. Create your own list of situations, ordered from easiest to hardest, using the Practice Exposure Hierarchy for Non-acquiring below. After your hierarchy is developed, you will work with your clinician to decide which exposures you can do alone and which should be done with the help of a coach. To arrange non-shopping with a partner, work with your clinician to identify a willing and helpful family member or friend.

During your non-acquiring exposures, record your discomfort level using a scale of 0 to 100 (where 0 equals no discomfort and 100 equals the most discomfort you've ever felt) about every 10 minutes, or whenever you notice a change in discomfort. This can be done on a small card carried in your hand or by telling your coach or partner. You will be surprised by how the intensity of the urge and the discomfort associated with it go away fairly quickly. Figure 5.1 is a graph of some data we collected on a non-shopping trip with some clients.

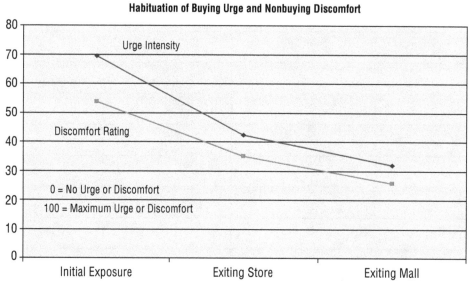

Figure 5.1

Reduction in urges to acquire and discomfort ratings for 8 people with acquiring problems during a non-shopping exercise at an International OCD Foundation workshop.

Practice Exposure Hierarchy for Non-acquiring

Situation   **Discomfort rating**

1. _____

2. _____

3. _____

4. _____

5. _____

6. _____

7. _____

8. _____

9. _____

10. _____

Alternative Sources of Enjoyment and Coping

If shopping or acquiring has become one of your main sources of enjoyment, it is important to find replacement activities that you find equally fun and fulfilling. For example, what would you like to do instead of going to flea markets or yard sales on Saturday? Use problem-solving skills (Chapter 6) to brainstorm a short list of likely alternatives, especially activities that can be done spontaneously, alone and/or in the company of friends, and inside and/or out of your home. Create your own list of alternative activities using the My Pleasurable Alternative Activities list below. List the activity and rate how pleasurable you expect it to be using a scale from 0 to 10.

Cognitive Strategies

As for work on sorting clutter, cognitive strategies provide excellent methods for changing thinking and beliefs, and helping you cope effectively with non-acquiring exposures. The following methods are designed specifically to help you resist urges to acquire. Be sure to use them during office sessions while planning non-acquiring exposures as well as during the actual acquiring situation.

Faulty Thinking Styles

Observing how your thoughts contribute to your acquiring problem is one of the most effective ways to change your behavior. Identifying patterns in your thinking helps you learn to avoid mental traps that are caused by your erroneous thoughts. The Problematic Thinking Styles list shown here will help you identify thinking errors when they occur during your office visits, as well as when completing your homework assignments.

1. *All-or-nothing thinking*—Black-or-white thinking that does not allow for shades of gray (moderation). It is exemplified by extreme words like *most, everything,* and *nothing,* and often accompanies perfectionistic standards.

   "This is the most beautiful teapot I have ever seen and I must have it."
   "I won't remember anything about this if I can't bring home this reminder."
   "I'll never have another opportunity if I don't get this now."

2. *Overgeneralization*—Generalization from a single event to all situations by using words such as *always* or *never*

   "I will never find this again if I don't get it now."

My Pleasurable Alternative Activities

Activity   **Pleasure Rating**

1. _____

2. _____

3. _____

4. _____

5. _____

6. _____

7. _____

8. _____

9. _____

10. _____

11. _____

12. _____

13. _____

14. _____

15. _____

"Whenever I see a bargain, I should take advantage of it
because I have always regretted not getting those pink shoes
I wanted when I was 12."
"They'll think I'm a fool for passing this up."
"If I don't get it now, I'll find out later that I really needed it."
"This might be useful, so I better get it because it could be
really important."

3. *Jumping to conclusions*—Negative interpretations (e.g., predicting that things will turn out badly) without facts to support them

"I won't remember this if I don't buy it."
"I better get this because as soon as I don't, I'll wish I had."
"I must get this newspaper because it has some useful
information I am certain to need eventually and can't find
elsewhere."

4. *Catastrophizing*—Exaggerating the importance of outcomes or items

"If I don't have this information when I need it, that's when
I'll find out it could have saved my husband's life."
"I'll fall apart if I don't get this."
"If I don't buy it now, I'll regret it forever."
"I'll never forgive myself."

5. *Discounting the positive*—Thinking that positive experiences don't count

"Resisting the urge to pick up literature at a conference doesn't
count because this was minor compared with the need to
spend less money buying things."
"I didn't do a good enough job on this; others could have done
it better."

6. *Emotional reasoning*—Allowing emotions to overwhelm logical reasoning; confusing facts with feelings

"It bothers me to leave this without getting it, so I must need it."
"I don't want to disappoint the salesman, so I'm sure I'll find
I need this."

"It seems like there must be something important in this paper. I better get it."

7. *Moral reasoning*—"Should" statements, including "must," "ought," and "have to," accompanied by guilt and frustration. Perfectionistic standards often play a role here.

"I really should be able to find any information I need at any time."
"I really should have the most up-to-date information about health problems in case something happens."
"My home should be very neat and tidy, just like other people's homes."

8. *Labeling*—Attaching a negative label to oneself or others; also an extreme form of all-or-nothing thinking

"I'd feel stupid if I didn't have the right information in case someone needed it."
"I'm an idiot; I should have got that when it was cheaper."
"I can't remember what I read last week. I'm so stupid."
"I'm a loser."
"I'm a fool."
"I'm a failure."
"He's an idiot."

9. *Underestimating oneself*—Underestimating personal ability to cope with adversity and stress

"If I don't get this, I won't be able to handle it and I'll have to come back for it later."
"If I do get rid of this, I'm sure I'll come back later to get it."

10. *Overestimating oneself*—Assuming greater capability to accomplish a task than is reasonable

"I'll be able to resist picking up all that free literature, so I'll just go check it out."
"I can clean this all up in a day or two."

Downward Arrow Method

The downward arrow method is a cognitive technique that helps clarify thoughts and beliefs. Your clinician may have already done this with you in session. Select an item that would provoke moderate discomfort when you think about not acquiring it and list it on the Downward Arrow Form here. How distressed, on a scale of 0 to 100, do you feel about not acquiring this item?

Defining Need Versus Want

Follow these steps for evaluating need versus want. Select an item you are considering acquiring and rate your need for it on a scale from 0 (don't need it at all) to 10 (need it very much) by circling the appropriate number on the scale.

Need to Acquire Scale

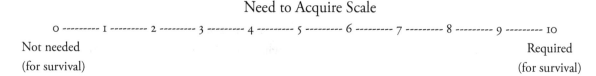

0 --------- 1 --------- 2 --------- 3 --------- 4 --------- 5 --------- 6 --------- 7 --------- 8 --------- 9 --------- 10

Not needed   Required

(for survival)   (for survival)

Next, rate how much you want to acquire the item on the following scale by circling the appropriate number on the scale.

Want to Acquire Scale

0 --------- 1 --------- 2 --------- 3 --------- 4 --------- 5 --------- 6 --------- 7 --------- 8 --------- 9 --------- 10

Don't want   Desperate

                                                    for

If you rate your need for the item as fairly low (<5) but your rating of want for the item as moderately high (>5), you are probably experiencing a conflict between your wants and your actual needs. The following questions can help you reduce your wish to acquire the items. Ask yourself the following questions and then reevaluate your desire for the item:

- How much do you need to get this item?

- Would you die without it?

- Would your safety be impaired without it?

Downward Arrow Form

Item: _____

In thinking about not acquiring or getting rid of (discarding, recycling, selling, giving away) this, what thoughts occur to you?

_____

_____

_____

If you didn't acquire or got rid of this, what do you think would happen?

_____

_____

_____

If this were true, why would it be so upsetting? (What would it mean to you? Why would that be so bad?)

_____

_____

_____

If that were true, what's so bad about that?

_____

_____

_____

What's the worst part about that?

_____

_____

_____

What does that mean about *you?*

_____

_____

_____

Additional copies of the Downward Arrow Form can be found in the Appendix.

- Would your health be jeopardized?

- Must you have this for your work?

- Do you need it for financial purposes (e.g., tax or insurance records)?

- Is there some other reason why you need the item?

- Do you actually *need* this or would it just be *convenient* to have it?

Homework

- Carry your Acquiring Questions Form during outings, and possibly laminate it.

- Develop a list of potential practice situations using the Practice Exposure Hierarchy for Non-acquiring; order these from least to most difficult.

- Select non-acquiring situations you can practice before the next session; keep a record of these for discussion in session. Record the context and items for each situation.

- Notice thoughts during practice outings to identify thinking errors.

- Use thinking strategies that seem most helpful during non-acquiring practices (for example: advantages/ disadvantages, need versus want scales, acquiring questions).

- Plan enjoyable activities as alternatives to acquiring during the week and record the expected and actual degree of pleasure experienced during these.

Chapter 6   *Skills Training*

Goals

- To learn effective problem-solving skills

- To develop organizing skills

- To create and implement a Personal Organizing Plan

- To learn strategies for organizing paper and how to create a filing system

Remember to use the Personal Session Form to make notes about your agenda, points you want to recall from the session, homework assignments, and any topics you want to discuss next time. Copies of the form are included in the Appendix.

Problem-Solving

Learning to solve problems and to categorize, file, and store items out of sight is essential for successful resolution of hoarding. Some simple steps for problem solving are shown in Table 6.1.

Problem-solving is appropriate whenever you are having trouble accomplishing a task or dealing with a difficult situation. These steps may seem obvious, but it is easy to omit one or more of them and to cut a task short. Ask your therapist to help you avoid this pitfall by making sure you follow all the steps systematically, especially the step in which you generate as many solutions as possible. Be careful not to make judgments about these ideas while you generate them. This step asks you to be creative—an important key to finding good solutions.

Table 6.1 Problem-Solving Steps

1. Define the problem and contributing factors.
2. Generate as many solutions as possible.
3. Evaluate the solutions and select one or two that seem feasible.
4. Break the solution into manageable steps.
5. Implement the steps.
6. Evaluate the outcome.
7. If necessary, repeat the process until a good solution is found.

Tracking Your Tasks

Setting priorities and keeping track of them in this *Workbook* are the keys to maintaining your focus on treatment. We have provided you with a Task List below to help you keep track of all your planned activities.

Organizing Skills for Objects

Your clinician will begin the organizing skills section of your treatment by helping your learn the best ways to organize your possessions. The first step is to define a few categories for items that will be removed from your home and then work on categorizing items that you will save.

Unwanted Items

The following categories are likely to be the main choices for how to dispose of any items you would like to remove from your home:

- Trash

- Recycle

- Donate (e.g., charities, library, friends, family)

- Sell (e.g., yard sale, bookstore, consignment shop, Internet sales)

- Undecided

You will work with your clinician to develop an action plan for how and when to remove items in each of these categories.

Task List

Priority Rating	Task	Date Put on List	Date Completed
A			
B			
C			

Additional copies of the Task List can be found in the Appendix.

Items to Save

The general organizing plan shown here includes a long list of categories of saved items (e.g., mail, photos, clothing, newspapers, office supplies) and typical locations where most people keep them, although this varies from person to person.

Organizing Plan

Categories for Saving	Locations for Storage
1. Mail and miscellaneous paper	File cabinets, drawers, processing pile
2. Magazines	Shelves, display, storage
3. Photos	Drawers, boxes
4. Newspapers	Recycle box
5. Clothing	Drawers, closets, laundry basket
6. Coats	Closets, rack
7. Boots and shoes	Closets, shoe rack
8. Books	Shelves, storage
9. Audio and videotapes	Shelves, drawers
10. Souvenirs	Display cabinets, drawers, storage
11. Decorative items	On display, storage
12. Gifts	Storage
13. Office supplies	Desk drawer, shelf, top of desk
14. Games	Shelves, cabinets
15. Hardware	Basement, garage, kitchen drawer
16. Furniture	Placed in room, storage
17. Empty containers	Cupboards, basement, garage
18. Food	Refrigerator, cupboard, pantry
19. Kitchen utensils	Drawers, containers

Categories for Saving	Locations for Storage
20. Pots, pans, and dishes	Cupboards, on hooks
21. Linens	Dining room cabinet, linen closet
22. Toiletries	Bathroom shelves, cabinets, drawers
23. Cleaning products	Kitchen, bath or laundry cabinets
24. Cleaning tools	Closet
25. Garden and yard tools	Garage, basement
26. Recreation equipment	Garage, basement, attic, closet
27. Paint and equipment	Garage, basement
28. Pet food and equipment	Closet, cupboard
29. Handicrafts	Cabinet, shelf, basement

The blank Personal Organizing Plan below will help you determine what kinds of items clutter your home and need to be classified and organized. From the general organizing plan, choose and list a category for each item in your home that needs to be categorized in the left-hand column of your Personal Organizing Plan and write down the final location (room, piece of furniture, and so forth) where each item belongs. You must eventually have an appropriate storage/filing location for all your things. Filing cabinets, bookshelves, and other storage furnishings may be needed to help you get organized.

The Preparing for Organizing Form will help you decide what preparations are needed before you are able to begin major sorting tasks. Begin by selecting a room and determining what types of objects you have within that space. Think through how you would store these objects when you have finished sorting them all. Do you need bookcases, file folders, a filing cabinet, hangers for a closet, plastic bins, or any other storage strategies? Record these items on the form so you can obtain them before you start.

After the organizing plan, necessary equipment, and storage locations are in place, you can begin sorting your things using the decision tree shown in Figure 6.1.

Personal Organizing Plan

Target area: _____

Item category	Final location
1. _____	_____
2. _____	_____
3. _____	_____
4. _____	_____
5. _____	_____
6. _____	_____
7. _____	_____
8. _____	_____
9. _____	_____
10. _____	_____
11. _____	_____
12. _____	_____
13. _____	_____
14. _____	_____
15. _____	_____
16. _____	_____
17. _____	_____
18. _____	_____
19. _____	_____
20. _____	_____

Additional copies of the Personal Organizing Plan can be found in the Appendix.

Preparing for Organizing Form

Room selection: _____

Target area or type of object selected: _____

Things I need to do to prepare for organizing:

1. _____

   _____

2. _____

   _____

3. _____

   _____

4. _____

   _____

5. _____

   _____

6. _____

   _____

Suggested tasks include:

- Getting boxes or storage containers

- Getting labels for boxes

- Clearing space for interim and final destinations

- Clearing space for sorting

- Scheduling times for working

Additional copies of the Preparing for Organizing Form can be found in the Appendix.

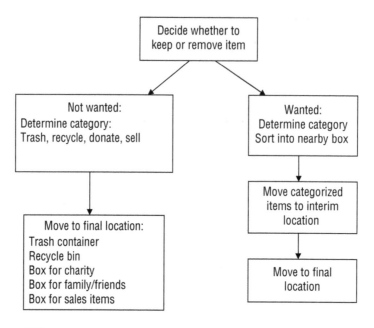

Figure 6.1
Decimion Tree for Sorting

Skills for Organizing Paper

People who hoard often mix important and unimportant things, such as checks and bills mixed with grocery store flyers and newspapers. To help you organize paperwork, it is crucial to set up a filing system for bills and documents, as well as places to store other papers like informational materials, upcoming events, travel information, pictures, and so on. Establishing a filing system early on helps with the sorting of items in each room. You might want to consult with friends or family members who seem to be well organized for ideas and suggestions.

Deciding how to file your paperwork can be difficult. We provide some suggestions in the following list.

How Long to Save Paper

Keep for One Month

- Credit card receipts

- Sales receipts for minor purchases

- Withdrawal and deposit slips. Toss after you've checked them against your monthly bank statement.

Keep for One Year

- Paycheck stubs/direct deposit receipts

- Monthly bank, credit card, brokerage, mutual fund, and retirement account statements

Keep for Six Years

- W-2 forms, 1099s, and other "guts" of your tax returns

- Year-end credit card statements, and brokerage and mutual fund summaries

Keep Indefinitely

- Tax returns

- Receipts for major purchases

- Real estate and residence records

- Wills and trusts

Keep in a Safety Deposit Box

- Birth and death certificates

- Marriage licenses

- Insurance policies

Review the Filing Paper Form below to determine which of the categories listed are relevant for your own filing system.

Like you did earlier, you may complete another Personal Organizing Plan, but this time, do it for all your paper items (Personal Organizing Plan for Papers below). A few simple general organizing rules like those listed in Figure 6.2 can be photocopied from this *Workbook* and posted on your refrigerator door (Anne Goodwin, 2006, April, personal communication).

Filing Paper Form

- Addresses and phone numbers
- Archives: wills, insurance policies, other important papers
- Articles (unread; after reading, put in a file of their own [e.g., Garden, Cooking])
- Automobile
- Catalogs
- Checking account(s)
- Computer
- Correspondence
- Coupons
- Diskettes
- Entertainment
- Financial
    - Credit cards
    - Bank statements
    - Retirement
    - Savings account(s)
    - Stocks
- Humor
- Individuals (by name); one file for each household member
- Instruction manuals/warranties
- Medical
- Personal/sentimental
- Photographs (before they get installed in an album)
- Product information
- Restaurants
- School papers
- Services
- Stamps
- Stationery
- Taxes
- Things-to-do lists
- Things to file (things that have to be reviewed)
- Calendar items (reminders for that specific month)
- Trips/vacation information

Things I need to get for filing paper:

1. _____

_____

2. _____

_____

3. _____

_____

4. _____

_____

Suggested items include

- File folders
- Hanging files
- Filing cabinets
- Labels
- Desk organizer

Personal Organizing Plan for Papers

Target area: _____

Item category	Final location
1. _____	_____
2. _____	_____
3. _____	_____
4. _____	_____
5. _____	_____
6. _____	_____
7. _____	_____
8. _____	_____
9. _____	_____
10. _____	_____
11. _____	_____
12. _____	_____
13. _____	_____
14. _____	_____
15. _____	_____
16. _____	_____
17. _____	_____
18. _____	_____
19. _____	_____
20. _____	_____

If you take it out, put it back.

If you open it, close it.

If you throw it down, pick it up.

If you take it off, hang it up.

If you use it, clean it up.

Figure 6.2
General Organizing Rules

Homework

- Practice problem-solving steps for a problem identified during one of your sessions.

- Call charities and sales outlets to make plans to remove unwanted possessions.

- Fill out the Preparing for Organizing Form and complete the selected tasks before your next session.

- Complete the Personal Organizing Plan and use it to sort items in the current target work area and move them to their intended location.

- Complete the Personal Organizing Plan for Papers.

- Identify appropriate filing space for paper and non-paper items, and assemble necessary materials.

- Generate file categories, label file folders, and put papers in an interim or final location for filing.

- Collect a few days' worth of mail and bring it to your session to sort with your clinician.

- Bring to your session any items for discussion that you could not decide on or categorize at home.

- Continue, during your session, any other tasks begun at home.

- Develop a plan for using cleared spaces and for keeping them clear of new clutter.

Chapter 7

Making Decisions About Saving and Discarding

Goals

- To conduct a thought listing exercise
- To develop a thought listing exercise hierarchy
- To participate in decision-making exercises regarding saving/discarding

Remember to use the Personal Session Form to make notes about your agenda, points you want to recall from the session, homework assignments, and any topics you want to discuss next time. Copies of the form are included in the Appendix.

Avoidance and Habituation

Think back to your model of hoarding and the role of avoidance. As you will recall, much of the problem in hoarding is associated with avoiding the unpleasantness associated with making decisions to get rid of possessions. In this chapter we will begin to tackle that avoidance.

The most effective way to overcome fear and discomfort is to expose yourself to situations you usually avoid because they make you feel uncomfortable. The more often you put yourself in a situation that is uncomfortable for you, the more you will get used to it, and the less discomfort you will feel. This process is called *habituation*. It is similar to the process that happens when you move to a new place near a train track or subway. At first, the sound bothers you, but after a while, you get used to it. Eventually, you hardly notice sounds that used to bother you a lot. Don't worry, we will begin slowly.

Some people habituate slowly, others quickly, and others have up-and-down reactions that gradually reduce over time. The habituation graph illustrated in Figure 7.1 shows a gradual drop in discomfort as exposure to an uncomfortable situation continues.

Your clinician will probably have done this exercise with you in your last session. It is a very simple exercise that can have a big impact on the way you make decisions about discarding. In this exercise choose a possession that you will have some trouble discarding. Don't choose something that is easy to get rid of, because the exercise won't have much meaning. Then rate how much distress you anticipate you would feel if you were to discard it. You do not have to discard it, only to consider it. Then indicate how long you think that distress will last. Turn to the Thought Listing Exercise Form shown below and record the item and your ratings.

At this point, you should have a pretty clear sense of how difficult discarding this item would be. Now, your task is to spend the next 4 minutes describing this item. Describe your thoughts out loud so you can hear yourself talk. Make mental notes about the thoughts that come to mind. Later on, you can record them on the Thought Listing Exercise Form.

At the end of the 4 minutes, make a decision about whether to keep or discard the item. If you decide to keep the item, use the organizing skills you developed earlier and put it where it belongs. If you decided

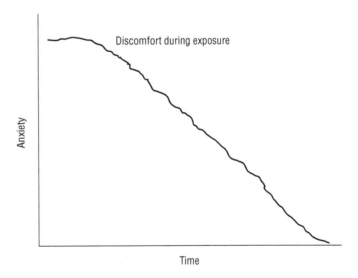

Figure 7.1
Habituation Graph

Thought Listing Exercise Form

Initials _____   Date _____

Selected Item:

Anticipated Distress Rating (from 0=none to 100=maximum): _____

Predicted Duration of Distress: _____

Thoughts about Discarding: _____

Discarding Decision (circle):   *Discard or Keep*

Distress rating after Decision: _____

Distress rating after 5 minutes: _____

Distress rating after 10 minutes: _____

Distress rating after 15 minutes: _____

Distress rating after 20 minutes: _____

Distress rating after 25 minutes: _____

Distress rating after 30 minutes: _____

Notes from Exercise:

_____

_____

_____

_____

_____

_____

Additional Copies of the Thought Listing Exercise Form can be found in the appendices.

to get rid of it, move it to the trash or out of the living area. Make a rating of your level of distress on the Thought Listing Exercise Form, and make new ratings every 5 minutes for the next half hour. Bring your completed form to the next session to discuss with your clinician.

Generating Questions

After trying the thought listing exercise a few times, think about thoughts or questions that make a difference to you as you decide whether to save or get rid of each item. Select a few that seem especially useful and write these on the Questions About Possessions Form. Ask yourself these questions for each item you sort. Below are some examples our clients have found useful. Some of these questions are similar to the ones listed in chapter 5 for making decisions about acquiring.

- How many do I already have and is that enough?
- Do I have enough time to use, review, or read it?
- Have I used this during the past year?
- Do I have a specific plan to use this item within a reasonable time frame?
- Does this fit with my own values and needs?
- How does this compare with the things I value highly?
- Does this just seem important because I'm looking at it now?
- Is it current?
- Is it of good quality, accurate, and/or reliable?
- Is it easy to understand?
- Would I buy it again if I didn't already own it?
- Do I really need it?
- Could I get it again if I found I really needed it?
- Do I have enough space for this?
- Will not having this help me solve my hoarding problem?

Questions About Possessions Form

_____

_____

_____

_____

_____

_____

_____

_____

_____

_____

_____

_____

_____

_____

A copy of the Questions About Possessions Form can be found in the Appendix.

Rules for Saving

Sorting can be facilitated by creating a set of general rules that remove the necessity of making decisions about each separate object. Work with your clinician to generate rules you will find useful in determining when to discard. For example, items not used during the past year and those with more than one copy could be discarded. Another example is to get rid of all items of clothing and jewelry that are not flattering to you or that you would not choose to buy now. It is also important to have rules for recycling, selling, and giving away items. Record your rules on the My Rules for Saving Form here.

My Rules for Saving Form

1. _____

2. _____

3. _____

4. _____

5. _____

Imagined Discarding

For possessions that seem just too hard to get rid of, your clinician may recommend imagined discarding. Prolonged imagined exposures of this sort can help you prepare for more difficult tasks, especially if you are fearful of sorting and possibly discarding your possessions.

Begin by selecting a difficult situation or behavior, like letting go of something moderately difficult—something you like but don't love. You can use imagined exposure to challenge your beliefs as well. For instance, you can imagine losing the information in a magazine and think about why that worries you. When you have a situation in mind, try to get a vivid picture of as many details as possible, including sounds, sights, smells, touch—use all your senses. Focus on your emotional reactions to letting go as well, such as fear, guilt, or sadness. Imagine picking up the object, dropping it into the trash, and putting the trash outside for pickup. Maintain the image until the emotion begins to drain away. Keep in mind that you want to imagine the worst part of the situation, the part with the most distress. Doing this actually helps you habituate faster.

Developing Your Thought Listing Exercise Hierarchy

Your clinician will help you develop a hierarchy of increasingly difficult decision-making situations. For example, discarding papers

Exposure Hierarchy Form

	Type of item	Location	Discomfort rating
1.	_____	_____	_____
2.	_____	_____	_____
3.	_____	_____	_____
4.	_____	_____	_____
5.	_____	_____	_____
6.	_____	_____	_____
7.	_____	_____	_____
8.	_____	_____	_____
9.	_____	_____	_____
10.	_____	_____	_____

with unidentified phone numbers may be easy for you, whereas getting rid of newspapers may be more difficult. Create your own list of items and locations in your home, ordered from easiest to hardest. Use the Exposure Hierarchy Form included here. Although you will undoubtedly experience some discomfort while you sort your things, the intent is gradually to increase your tolerance for making decisions and getting rid of items.

After creating your hierarchy, start sorting at home and in the office. You can begin with the items that will cause the least discomfort, the "easiest" items on your list.

Behavioral Experiments

Behavioral experiments provide opportunities to test some of your beliefs about possessions and how letting go of them actually affects you. They begin with a brief description of the experiment, followed

Behavioral Experiment Form

Initials: _____   Date: _____

1. Behavioral experiment to be completed: _____

   _____

   _____

2. What do you predict (are afraid) will happen? _____

   _____

   _____

3. How strongly do you believe this will happen (0–100%) _____

   _____

4. Initial discomfort (0–100) _____

5. What actually happened? _____

   _____

   _____

   _____

6. Final discomfort (0–100) _____

7. Did your predictions come true? _____

8. What conclusions do you draw from this experiment? _____

   _____

   _____

   _____

   _____

by what you predict will happen. The prediction is usually your reason for saving the item. For example, "I won't be able to stand it if I throw this magazine away." Next rate how strongly you believe the prediction and then indicate your rating of initial discomfort on a scale from 0 = none to 100 = maximum. At this point, go ahead and do the experiment (throw the object into the trash) and then record what actually happened, including how you felt, your level of discomfort, and your observations about whether your predictions came true. The conclusions you draw from the experiment are the final and most important part of the experiment. These conclusions tell you whether your prediction actually came true and whether your fears were worse than your actual experience.

A blank Behavioral Experiment Form is included here. Additional copies are included in the Appendix.

Structured Cleanouts

We generally do not recommend cleanouts in hoarding cases, especially if they are forced. However, at some point you and your therapist may want to do a structured cleanout, especially if your home has a large amount of clutter and many hands will make the work easier. These events are usually day-long affairs during which family members, friends, volunteers, or cleaning crews help you clear out the clutter based on the rules you have established. It is best to do this after you have had some experience with the exercises described in this chapter and have developed a clear set of rules that work well for you because they help you get rid of many items but save the really important ones. Cleanouts take careful planning, coordination, and written rules that everyone follows. Cleanouts are a form of extended exposure and should be planned and accomplished with the help of your clinician.

Homework

- Repeat the thought listing exercise with three items at home.

- Imagine getting rid of items before actually discarding/recycling them.

- Conduct a planned behavioral experiment to test a specific hypothesis, especially about the discomfort and consequences of parting with possessions.

- Take home items to be saved from the thought listing exercise and store them where they belong.

- Bring in additional items (e.g., photos, mail, items from a particular area) to office appointments for sorting and decision-making exposures.

- Make arrangements for trash removal and, in the case of a major cleanout, for dumpster delivery and removal.

Chapter 8

Changing Beliefs: Thinking Your Way Out of the Hoarding Box

Goals

- To work with your clinician to identify errors in your thinking

- To learn techniques to change beliefs and use them during your decision-making sessions

Remember to use the Personal Session Form to make notes about your agenda, points you want to recall from the session, homework assignments, and any topics you want to discuss next time. Copies of the form are included in the Appendix.

Errors in Thinking

Because of their importance, here we revisit the problematic thinking styles discussed earlier. Identifying patterns in your thinking helps you learn to avoid mental traps that are caused by faulty thoughts. The Problematic Thinking Styles list shown here will help you identify thinking errors when they occur as you are making decisions about saving and discarding. The examples here focus mostly on saving and discarding since we have already discussed faulty thinking in relation to acquiring in chapter 5.

Problematic Thinking Styles

1. *All-or-nothing thinking*—Black-or-white thinking that does not allow for shades of gray (moderation). It is exemplified by extreme words like *most, everything,* and *nothing,* and often accompanies perfectionistic standards.

"If I can't figure out the perfect place to put this, I should just leave it here."

"This must stay in sight or I'll forget it."

"I can't get rid of this until I read and remember everything in this newspaper." "Now I will forget everything I know about this subject."

2. *Overgeneralization*—Generalization from a single event to all situations by using words such as *always* or *never*

"I will never find this if I move it."

"I'll need something just as soon as I don't have it anymore."

3. *Jumping to conclusions*—Negative interpretations (e.g., predicting that things will turn out badly) without facts to support them

"If I file this magazine article, I will never be able to find it."

"I won't remember this if I move it."

"My sister has offered to help me straighten up, but that's because she thinks I am a terrible person and she plans to throw away everything I own."

"If I throw away this magazine, I'll soon find that I need it."

"I must keep this newspaper because it has some useful information I am certain to need eventually."

4. *Catastrophizing*—Exaggerating the importance of an item and minimizing the ability to obtain needed information

"If I put this away and can't remember where I put it, it will be awful."

"If I don't have this information when I need it, that's when I'll find out it could have saved my husband's life."

"I'll fall apart if I don't have this."

"If I throw it away, I'll go crazy thinking about it."

"I'll never forgive myself."

5. *Discounting the positive*—Thinking that positive experiences don't count

"Creating a filing system doesn't count as progress because there is so much more to do."

"I didn't do a good enough job on this; others could have done it better."

"I got this cleared, but it hardly matters because the other rooms are still cluttered."

6. *Emotional reasoning*—Allowing emotions to determine logical reasoning; confusing facts with feelings

"It feels uncomfortable to put this out of sight, so I'll just leave it here."

"It bothers me to leave without buying it, so I must need it."

"If I feel uncomfortable about throwing this away, this means I should keep it."

"It seems like there must be something important in this paper. I better keep it."

7. *Moral reasoning*—"Should" statements, including "musts," "oughts," and "have to's," accompanied by guilt and frustration. Perfectionistic standards often play a role here.

"I really should be able to find any information I need at any time."

"I really should have the most up-to-date information about health problems in case something happens."

"My home should be very neat and tidy, just like other people's homes."

"I really should file this stuff."

8. *Labeling*—Attaching a negative label to oneself or others; also an extreme form of all-or-nothing thinking

"I can't find my electric bill. I'm an idiot."

"I'd feel stupid if I didn't have the right information in case someone needed it."

"I can't remember what I read last week. I'm so stupid."

"I'm a loser."

"I'm a fool."

"I'm a failure."

9. *Underestimating and overestimating oneself*—Underestimating or overestimating personal ability to cope with adversity and stress or capability to accomplish a task

"I'll never be able to organize all this."
"If I do get rid of this, I won't be able to handle it."
"I'll be able to organize my home during my (week-long) vacation."
"I'll be able to read all those newspapers eventually."

Cognitive Strategies

An important goal of this treatment program is to help you learn how to observe your own reactions and become aware of your thinking. After you and your clinician have identified the beliefs that maintain your hoarding problem, you will begin using the following cognitive strategies to change these beliefs.

Questions About Possessions

One way to help fix your errors in thinking is to pay attention to the reasons for *not* keeping an item. Review the Questions About Possessions from chapters 5 and 7 to determine which questions seem most useful. Keep these forms handy as you work on making decisions about your possessions.

Advantages and Disadvantages

Another strategy is to examine the advantages and disadvantages of keeping a particular item. People who hoard tend to focus on the immediate costs associated with discarding something, while ignoring the costs of saving all their possessions and the benefits of getting rid of them. Use the Advantages/Disadvantages Worksheet here to help you determine the personal advantages of keeping an item, followed by the disadvantages.

Advantages/Disadvantages Worksheet

Specify the item(s) under consideration: _____

Advantages (Benefits)	Disadvantages (Costs)
Of keeping/acquiring:	Of keeping/acquiring:
Of getting rid of item:	Of getting rid of item:

Downward Arrow Method

The downward arrow method discussed in chapter 5 is a cognitive technique that helps clarify thoughts and beliefs. Select an item that would be moderately hard to discard and list this on the Downward Arrow Form below.

Thought Record Form

During your practice exercises, you can work to change mistaken beliefs gradually by identifying alternative possibilities that make more sense to you. You can record these alternatives on the Thought Record Form below.

Defining Need Versus Want

Deciding the *true* value of a possession based on your own goals and rational thinking requires you to distinguish what you truly need from what you merely want. The Need Versus Want Scale below is useful for this purpose.

Select a current possession that would be moderately difficult but potentially appropriate for you to discard. Using the scales, record an initial rating of need and want for the particular item. Then, review the questions with your clinician to determine whether you change your ratings after thinking through the true value of possessions in relation to other important goals in your life.

Perfectionism Scale

If you are overly concerned about making mistakes, or your self-worth depends on how well you do things, it will be helpful to look at just how much of your life is driven by perfectionism. Use the Perfectionism Scale below to rate your discarding behaviors. But first, consider the following questions:

- Do your decisions have to be perfect?
- Do you have to get rid of things "just the right way"?
- Do you feel defective or bad when you make mistakes in discarding?

Try to rate each of your "letting go" or sorting decisions using the Perfectionism Scale.

Downward Arrow Form

Item: _____

In thinking about not acquiring or getting rid of (discarding, recycling, selling, giving away) this, what thoughts occur to you?

_____

_____

_____

If you didn't acquire or got rid of this, what do you think would happen?

_____

_____

_____

If this were true, why would it be so upsetting? (What would it mean to you? Why would that be so bad?)

_____

_____

_____

If that were true, what's so bad about that?

_____

_____

_____

What's the worst part about that?

_____

_____

_____

What does that mean about *you?*

_____

_____

_____

Thought Record Form

Initials: _____ Date: _____

Trigger situation	Thoughts	Emotions	Rational alternative	Outcome

Additional copies of the Thought Record Form can be found in the Appendix.

Need Versus Want Scales

Item: _____

Rate your need for the item on the following scale:

Need to Keep Scale

0 ---------- I ---------- 2 ---------- 3 ---------- 4 ---------- 5 ---------- 6 ---------- 7 ---------- 8 ---------- 9 ---------- IO

No need   Required

to survive

Rate how much you want or desire the item on this scale by circling a number on the Want to Acquire Scale.

Want to Keep Scale

0 ---------- I ---------- 2 ---------- 3 ---------- 4 ---------- 5 ---------- 6 ---------- 7 ---------- 8 ---------- 9 ---------- IO

Don't want   Desperate for

Now, let's consider the value of the item more carefully. To evaluate your true *need* for it, consider whether you need it for survival, safety, health, work, financial affairs, and/or recreation using the following questions:

- Would you die without it? _____

- Would your safety be impaired without it? _____

- Would your health be jeopardized without it? _____

- Is this critical to your work or employment? _____

- Is it essential for your financial records (e.g., tax or insurance records)? _____

Re-rate your need for the item using the Need to *Keep* Scale:

Need to Keep Scale

0 ---------- I ---------- 2 ---------- 3 ---------- 4 ---------- 5 ---------- 6 ---------- 7 ---------- 8 ---------- 9 ---------- IO

No need   Required

to survive

Need is different from want. To determine your *want* or wish for the item, think only about your urge to have it, regardless of actual need. Consider the following questions:

- Do you keep this because you like it? How much do you actually look at it?

_____

_____

_____

Are you keeping it for sentimental reasons? Is this the best way to remember?

_____

_____

_____

How much do you actually use it now? If you plan to use it soon, would you bet money on this?

_____

_____

_____

Do you keep this for emotional comfort or vulnerability? Does it really protect you?

_____

_____

_____

Does it offer information or opportunity? How real and important is that?

_____

_____

_____

Now, re-rate how much you want or desire the item using the following Want to Acquire Scale:

Want to Keep Scale

0 ---------- 1 ---------- 2 ---------- 3 ---------- 4 ---------- 5 ---------- 6 ---------- 7 ---------- 8 --------- 9 --------- 10

Don't want   Desperate for

Comments and conclusions: _____

_____

_____

_____

_____

_____

_____

Perfectionism Scale

0 ------------- 1 ---------- 2 ---------- 3 ---------- 4 ---------- 5 ---------- 6 ---------- 7 ---------- 8 --------- 9 --------- 10

Defective	Average	Perfect
Wrong	Okay	Exactly right

Valuing Your Time

Are you saving things until you have more time to deal with them? If so, ask yourself some pointed questions:

1. Do you have more reading material (e.g., newspapers, magazines) than you have time to read?

   - If so, do you really want to spend the time necessary to read them?

   - What other parts of your life will you miss or will suffer by doing so?
   - How does this fit with your values and goals?

2. Do you have more _____ (fill in the blank) than you can possibly use?

   - If so, do you really want to spend the time necessary to deal with them?

   - What other parts of your life will you miss or will suffer by doing so?
   - How does this fit with your values and goals?

Homework

- Review the Problematic Thinking Styles list to identify some that occur during the coming week. Identify alternative thinking that avoids the error.

- Apply the Questions About Possessions while sorting.

- Use the Advantages/Disadvantages Worksheet to evaluate the advantages and disadvantages of keeping a particular item.

- Complete the Downward Arrow Form to identify beliefs associated with letting go of possessions.

- Use the Thought Record Form to evaluate the accuracy of current reasons for saving and consider alternative ones.

- Use the Need Versus Want and Perfectionism scales during sorting at home when decision-making seems difficult.

- Calculate the time cost associated with keeping objects.

Chapter 9   *Maintaining Your Gains*

Goals

- To review your progress up to this point

- To develop strategies to continue working on your hoarding problem in the future

- To identify the treatment methods that worked best for you

- To anticipate and develop strategies for coping with setbacks and lapses

Remember to use the Personal Session Form to make notes about your agenda, points you want to recall from the session, homework assignments, and any topics you want to discuss next time. Copies of the form are included in the Appendix.

Reviewing Your Progress

During your final sessions with your clinician, you will review your progress up to this point and discuss how to plan for your future. You may not yet have completely achieved your goal of freedom from compulsive hoarding problems, but if you have made some progress, it is very likely that you can continue to do so. Nonetheless, changing habits takes time and you will need to work on the remaining clutter in your home and your urges to acquire for some time to come until your new habits become second nature.

Measuring Your Progress

At this stage of your treatment, your clinician will ask you to complete the assessment forms from chapter 2 to measure your progress. These

Table 9.1 Change in Hoarding Symptoms

Measure	Pre-test score	Post-test score (% improvement)	12-mo follow-up score (% improvement)
Hoarding Rating Scale	_____	_____ (%)	_____ (%)
Saving Inventory–Revised—Total score	_____	_____ (%)	_____ (%)
SI-R Clutter	_____	_____ (%)	_____ (%)
SI-R Difficulty Discarding	_____	_____ (%)	_____ (%)
SI-R Acquisition	_____	_____ (%)	_____ (%)
Clutter Image Rating	_____	_____ (%)	_____ (%)
Saving Cognitions Inventory	_____	_____ (%)	_____ (%)
SCI Emotional Attachment	_____	_____ (%)	_____ (%)
SCI Control	_____	_____ (%)	_____ (%)
SCI Responsibility	_____	_____ (%)	_____ (%)
SCI Memory	_____	_____ (%)	_____ (%)
Activities of Daily Living for Hoarding	_____	_____ (%)	_____ (%)
Safety Questions	_____	_____ (%)	_____ (%)
Home Environment Index	_____	_____ (%)	_____ (%)

include the following: Hoarding Rating Scale, Saving Inventory–Revised, Clutter Image Rating, Saving Cognitions Inventory, Activities of Daily Living for Hoarding (ADL-H), Safety Questions, and Home Environment Index. Completing these one more time helps you and your clinician see how much change has occurred in all areas related to hoarding (Table 9.1). The assessment forms can be scored using the score key in the Appendix.

Continuing Treatment on Your Own

It is likely that your therapist will begin tapering your treatment sessions so they occur less frequently. During the weeks between sessions, you should begin a self-therapy plan. We suggest you schedule self-sessions on the same day and time slot when meetings with your clinician usually occurred. Schedule these sessions ahead of time and mark them on your calendar. Your clinician will work with you to develop a formal plan for your self-sessions. This will be the time to practice sorting and not acquiring using the methods you found most helpful during treatment.

Hoarding Rating Scale (HRS)

Client Initials: _____   Date: _____

1. Because of the clutter or number of possessions, how difficult is it for you to use the rooms in your home?

0 ----------- 1 ----------- 2 ----------- 3 ----------- 4 ----------- 5 ----------- 6 ----------- 7 ----------- 8
Not at all   Mild   Moderate   Severe   Extremely
Difficult   Difficult

2. To what extent do you have difficulty discarding (or recycling, selling, giving away) ordinary things that other people would get rid of?

0 ----------- 1 ----------- 2 ----------- 3 ----------- 4 ----------- 5 ----------- 6 ----------- 7 ----------- 8
Not at all   Mild   Moderate   Severe   Extremely
Difficult   Difficult

3. To what extent do you currently have a problem with collecting free things or buying more things than you need or can use or can afford? [Use the scale below]

0 ----------- 1 ----------- 2 ----------- 3 ----------- 4 ----------- 5 ----------- 6 ----------- 7 ----------- 8
No problem   Extreme

0 = no problem
2 = mild problem, occasionally (less than weekly) acquires items not needed,
    or acquires a few unneeded items
4 = moderate, regularly (once or twice weekly) acquires items not needed, or
    acquires some unneeded items
6 = severe, frequently (several times per week) acquires items not needed,
    or acquires many unneeded items
8 = extreme, very often (daily) acquires items not needed, or acquires large
    numbers of unneeded items

4. To what extent do you experience emotional distress because of clutter, difficulty discarding or problems with buying or acquiring things?

0 ----------- 1 ----------- 2 ----------- 3 ----------- 4 ----------- 5 ----------- 6 ----------- 7 ----------- 8
None/   Mild   Moderate   Severe   Extreme
Not at all

5. To what extent do you experience impairment in your life (daily routine, job / school, social activities, family activities, financial difficulties) because of clutter, difficulty discarding, or problems with buying or acquiring things?

0 ----------- 1 ----------- 2 ----------- 3 ----------- 4 ----------- 5 ----------- 6 ----------- 7 ----------- 8
None/   Mild   Moderate   Severe   Extreme
Not at all

Saving Inventory – Revised

Client Initials: _____   Date: _____

For each question below, circle the number that corresponds most closely to your experience DURING THE PAST WEEK.

0 --------------- 1 ------------------ 2 ---------------- 3 ---------------- 4

None	A little	A moderate amount	Most/Much	Almost All/ Complete

1. How much of the living area in your home is cluttered with possessions? (Consider the amount of clutter in your kitchen, living room, dining room, hallways, bedrooms, bathrooms, or other rooms).   0   1   2   3   4

2. How much control do you have over your urges to acquire possessions?   0   1   2   3   4

3. How much of your home does clutter prevent you from using?   0   1   2   3   4

4. How much control do you have over your urges to save possessions?   0   1   2   3   4

5. How much of your home is difficult to walk through because of clutter?   0   1   2   3   4

For each question below, circle the number that corresponds most closely to your experience DURING THE PAST WEEK.

0 --------------------- 1 ------------------ 2 ------------------ 3 ------------------ 4

Not at all	Mild	Moderate	Considerable/ Severe	Extreme

6. To what extent do you have difficulty throwing things away?   0   1   2   3   4

7. How distressing do you find the task of throwing things away?   0   1   2   3   4

8. To what extent do you have so many things that your room(s) are cluttered?   0   1   2   3   4

9. How distressed or uncomfortable would you feel if you could not acquire something you wanted?   0   1   2   3   4

10. How much does clutter in your home interfere with your social, work or everyday functioning? Think about things that you don't do because of clutter.   0   1   2   3   4

11. How strong is your urge to buy or acquire free things for which you have no immediate use?   0   1   2   3   4

For each question below, circle the number that corresponds most closely to your experience
DURING THE PAST WEEK:

0	1	2	3	4
Not at all	Mild	Moderate	Considerable/ Severe	Extreme

	0	1	2	3	4
12. To what extent does clutter in your home cause you distress?	0	1	2	3	4
13. How strong is your urge to save something you know you may never use?	0	1	2	3	4
14. How upset or distressed do you feel about your acquiring habits?	0	1	2	3	4
15. To what extent do you feel unable to control the clutter in your home?	0	1	2	3	4
16. To what extent has your saving or compulsive buying resulted in financial difficulties for you?	0	1	2	3	4

For each question below, circle the number that corresponds most closely to your experience
DURING THE PAST WEEK.

0	1	2	3	4
Never	Rarely	Sometimes/ Occasionally	Frequently/ Often	Very Often

	0	1	2	3	4
17. How often do you avoid trying to discard possessions because it is too stressful or time consuming?	0	1	2	3	4
18. How often do you feel compelled to acquire something you see? e.g., when shopping or offered free things?	0	1	2	3	4
19. How often do you decide to keep things you do not need and have little space for?	0	1	2	3	4
20. How frequently does clutter in your home prevent you from inviting people to visit?	0	1	2	3	4
21. How often do you actually buy (or acquire for free) things for which you have no immediate use or need?	0	1	2	3	4
22. To what extent does the clutter in your home prevent you from using parts of your home for their intended purpose? For example, cooking, using furniture, washing dishes, cleaning, etc.	0	1	2	3	4
23. How often are you unable to discard a possession you would like to get rid of?	0	1	2	3	4

Clutter Image Rating

Date: _____

Using the 3 series of pictures (CIR: Living Room, CIR: Kitchen, and CIR: Bedroom), please select the picture that best represents the amount of clutter for each of the rooms of your home. Put the number on the line below.

Please pick the picture that is closest to being accurate, even if it is not exactly right.

If your home does not have one of the rooms listed, just put NA for "not applicable" on that line.

Room	Number of closest corresponding picture (1–9)
Living Room	_____
Kitchen	_____
Bedroom #1	_____
Bedroom #2	_____

Also, please rate other rooms in your house that are affected by clutter on the lines below. Use the *CIR: Living Room* pictures to make these ratings.

Dining room   _____

Hallway   _____

Garage   _____

Basement   _____

Attic   _____

Car   _____

Other   _____   Please specify: _____

Scores above 3 in any room are cause for concern.

(*continued*)

Clutter Image Rating: Living Room

Please select the photo below that most accurately reflects the amount of clutter in your room.

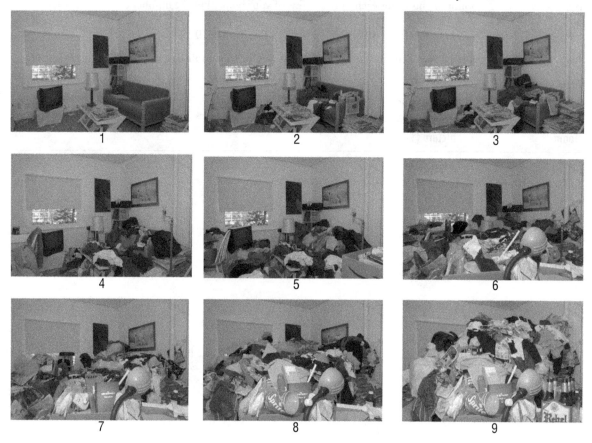

Figure 9.1

Clutter Image Rating Scale: Living Room

Clutter Image Rating Scale: Kitchen

Please select the photo below that most accurately reflects the amount of clutter in your room.

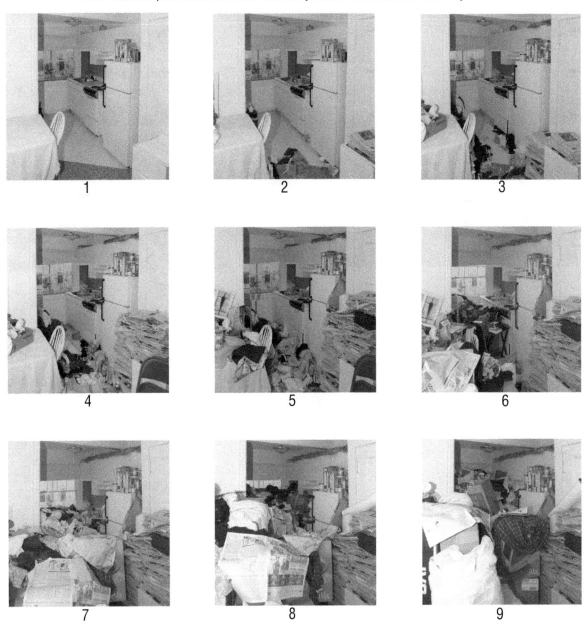

Figure 9.2

Clutter Image Rating Scale: Kitchen

Clutter Image Rating: Bedroom

Please select the photo that most accurately reflects the amount of clutter in your room.

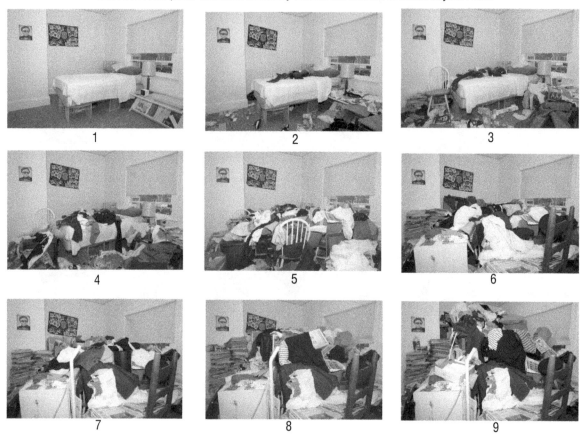

Figure 9.3

Clutter Image Rating Scale: Bedroom

Saving Cognitions Inventory

Date: _____

Use the following scale to indicate the extent to which you had each thought when you were deciding whether to throw something away DURING THE PAST WEEK. (If you did not try to discard anything in the past week, indicate how you would have felt if you had tried to discard.)

```
1 -------------- 2 -------------- 3 -------------- 4 -------------- 5 -------------- 6 -------------- 7
not at all                        sometimes                        very much
```

1. I could not tolerate it if I were to get rid of this.	1	2	3	4	5	6	7
2. Throwing this away means wasting a valuable opportunity.	1	2	3	4	5	6	7
3. Throwing away this possession is like throwing away a part of me.	1	2	3	4	5	6	7
4. Saving this means I don't have to rely on my memory.	1	2	3	4	5	6	7
5. It upsets me when someone throws something of mine away without my permission.	1	2	3	4	5	6	7
6. Losing this possession is like losing a friend.	1	2	3	4	5	6	7
7. If someone touches or uses this, I will lose it or lose track of it.	1	2	3	4	5	6	7
8. Throwing some things away would feel like abandoning a loved one.	1	2	3	4	5	6	7
9. Throwing this away means losing a part of my life.	1	2	3	4	5	6	7
10. I see my belongings as extensions of myself; they are part of who I am.	1	2	3	4	5	6	7
11. I am responsible for the well-being of this possession	1	2	3	4	5	6	7
12. If this possession may be of use to someone else, I am responsible for saving it for them.	1	2	3	4	5	6	7
13. This possession is equivalent to the feelings I associate with it.	1	2	3	4	5	6	7
14. My memory is so bad I must leave this in sight or I'll forget about it.	1	2	3	4	5	6	7
15. I am responsible for finding a use for this possession.	1	2	3	4	5	6	7
16. Throwing some things away would feel like part of me is dying.	1	2	3	4	5	6	7
17. If I put this into a filing system, I'll forget about it completely.	1	2	3	4	5	6	7
18 I like to maintain sole control over my things.	1	2	3	4	5	6	7
19. I'm ashamed when I don't have something like this when I need it.	1	2	3	4	5	6	7
20. I must remember something about this, and I can't if I throw this away.	1	2	3	4	5	6	7
21. If I discard this without extracting all the important information from it, I will lose something.	1	2	3	4	5	6	7
22. This possession provides me with emotional comfort.	1	2	3	4	5	6	7
23. I love some of my belongings the way I love some people.	1	2	3	4	5	6	7
24. No one has the right to touch my possessions.	1	2	3	4	5	6	7

Activities of Daily Living for Hoarding (ADL-H)

Date: _____

Sometimes clutter in the home can prevent you from doing ordinary activities. For each of the following activities, please circle the number that best represents the degree of difficulty you experience in doing this activity because of the clutter or hoarding problem. If you have difficulty with the activity for other reasons (for example, unable to bend or move quickly due to physical problems), do not include this in your rating. Instead, rate only how much difficulty you would have **due to hoarding**. If the activity is not relevant to your situation (for example, you don't have laundry facilities or animals), circle Not Applicable (NA).

Activities affected by clutter or hoarding problem	Can do it easily	Can do it with a little difficulty	Can do it with moderate difficulty	Can do it with great difficulty	Unable to do	Not Applicable
1. Prepare food	1	2	3	4	5	NA
2. Use refrigerator	1	2	3	4	5	NA
3. Use stove	1	2	3	4	5	NA
4. Use kitchen sink	1	2	3	4	5	NA
5. Eat at table	1	2	3	4	5	NA
6. Move around inside the house	1	2	3	4	5	NA
7. Exit home quickly	1	2	3	4	5	NA
8. Use toilet	1	2	3	4	5	NA
9. Use bath/shower	1	2	3	4	5	NA
10. Use bathroom sink	1	2	3	4	5	NA
11. Answer door quickly	1	2	3	4	5	NA
12. Sit in sofa/chair	1	2	3	4	5	NA
13. Sleep in bed	1	2	3	4	5	NA
14. Do laundry	1	2	3	4	5	NA
15. Find important things (such as bills, tax forms, etc.)	1	2	3	4	5	NA

Safety Questions

Sometimes the clutter in your home can cause safety problems. Please circle the number below that best indicates how much of a problem you have with the following conditions in your home:

Safety problems in the home	None	A little	Somewhat/ moderate	Substantial	Severe
1. Is there structural damage to the floors, walls, roof, or other parts of your home?	1	2	3	4	5
2. Is your water not working?	1	2	3	4	5
3. Is your heat not working?	1	2	3	4	5
4. Does any part of your house pose a fire hazard? (stove covered with paper, flammable objects near the furnace, etc.)	1	2	3	4	5
5. Would medical emergency personnel have difficulty moving equipment through your home?	1	2	3	4	5
6. Are exits from your home blocked?	1	2	3	4	5
7. Is it unsafe to move up or down the stairs or along other walkways?	1	2	3	4	5

A score of 2 or above on any question is meaningful and needs attention.

Date: _____

Clutter and hoarding problems can sometimes lead to sanitation problems. Please circle the answer that best fits the current situation in the home.

To what extent are the following situations present in the home?

1. Fire hazard
   0 = No fire hazard
   1 = Some risk of fire (for example, lots of flammable material)
   2 = Moderate risk of fire (for example, flammable materials near heat source)
   3 = High of fire (for example, flammable materials near heat source; electrical hazards, etc.)

2. Moldy or rotten food
   0 = None
   1 = A few pieces of moldy or rotten food in kitchen
   2 = Some moldy or rotten food throughout kitchen
   3 = Large quantity of moldy or rotten food in kitchen and elsewhere

3. Dirty or clogged sink
   0 = Sink empty and clean
   1 = A few dirty dishes with water in sink
   2 = Sink full of water, possibly clogged
   3 = Sink clogged with evidence that it has overflowed onto counters, etc.

4. Standing water (in sink, tub, other container, basement, etc.)
   0 = No standing water
   1 = Some water in sink/tub
   2 = Water in several places, especially if dirty
   3 = Water in numerous places, especially if dirty

5. Human/animal waste/vomit
   0 = No human waste, animal waste, or vomit visible
   1 = Small amount of human or animal waste (e.g., unflushed toilet, on bathroom or other floor)
   2 = Moderate animal or human waste or vomit visible in more than one room
   3 = Substantial animal or human waste or vomit on floors or other surfaces

6. Mildew or mold
   0 = No mildew or mold detectable
   1 = Small amount of mildew or mold in limited amounts and expected places (for example, on edge of shower curtain or refrigerator seal)
   2 = Considerable, noticeable mildew or mold
   3 = Widespread mildew or mold on most surfaces

7. Dirty food containers
   0 = All dishes washed and put away
   1 = A few unwashed dishes
   2 = Many unwashed dishes
   3 = Almost all dishes are unwashed

8. Dirty surfaces (floors, walls, furniture, etc.)

   0 = Surfaces completely clean

   1 = A few spills, some dirt or grime

   2 = More than a few spills, may be a thin covering of dirt or grime in living areas

   3 = No surface is clean; dirt or grime covers everything

9. Piles of dirty or contaminated objects (bathroom tissue, hair, toilet paper, sanitary products, etc.)

   0 = No dirty or contaminated objects on floors, surfaces, etc.

   1 = Some dirty or contaminated objects present around trash cans or toilets

   2 = Many dirty or contaminated objects fill bathroom or area around trash cans

   3 = Dirty or contaminated objects cover the floors and surfaces in most rooms

10. Insects

    0 = No insects are visible

    1 = A few insects visible; cobwebs and/or insect droppings present

    2 = Many insects and droppings are visible; cobwebs in corners

    3 = Swarms of insects; high volume of droppings; many cobwebs on household items

11. Dirty clothes

    0 = Dirty clothes placed in hamper; none are lying around

    1 = Hamper is full; a few dirty clothes lying around

    2 = Hamper is overflowing; many dirty clothes lying around

    3 = Clothes cover the floor and many other surfaces (bed, chairs, etc.)

12. Dirty bed sheets/linens

    0 = Bed coverings very clean

    1 = Bed coverings relatively clean

    2 = Bed coverings dirty and in need of washing

    3 = Bed coverings very dirty and soiled

13. Odor of house

    0 = No odor

    1 = Slight odor

    2 = Moderate odor; may be strong in some parts of house

    3 = Strong odor throughout house

During the last month, how often did you (or someone in your home) do each of the following activities?

14. Do the dishes

    0 = Daily or every 2 days; 15 to 30 times per month

    1 = 1-2 times a week; 4 to 10 times per month

    3 = Every other week; 2 to 3 times per month

    3 = Rarely; 0 times per month

15. Clean the bathroom

    0 = Daily or every 2 days; more than 10 times per month

    1 = 1-2 times a week; 4 to 10 times per month

    2 = Every other week; 2 to 3 times per month

    3 = Never; 0 times per month

A score of 2 or above on any question warrants attention.

Also, consider finding or starting a Buried in Treasures Workshop with other people who also suffer from hoarding problems. This type of workshop is a time-limited structured group led by a non-clinician who is a peer or someone from the community who is familiar with hoarding and interested in facilitating a peer support group. Groups follow chapters in the book *Buried in Treasures* by Tolin, Frost, and Steketee, which is based on the same principles as this *Workbook*. Instructions for how to find or start a workshop can be found on the International OCD Foundation website: www.ocfoundation.org/hoarding.

Booster Sessions

Because many people need time to establish new habits, you and your clinician may wish to schedule two or three "booster sessions" a few months apart. These sessions can help you reconnect with your goals to eliminate hoarding problems and remind you of treatment techniques you may have forgotten. You and your clinician can decide whether you need these sessions and how far apart they should be. Or you might decide that you will call your clinician to set up a time whenever you feel you need a little more help.

Review Treatment Techniques

Reviewing the treatment techniques you've been using is a critical activity for preventing relapse and helps remind you of what you have learned. Begin by reviewing the compulsive hoarding and acquiring models developed early during your treatment (chapter 3). Ask yourself whether these models are still accurate and whether you would make any changes to them now.

Next, remind yourself of your original treatment goals by examining the Goals Form you completed during the treatment planning phase (chapter 4). Review what you have actually accomplished, including changes in symptoms (e.g., acquiring, clutter, ability to get rid of things) as well as skills developed (organizing, resisting impulses to acquire, problem-solving, managing attention).

Then, review the techniques you learned during therapy by going over your Personal Session Forms and other material in this *Workbook*. You can also review the list of treatment techniques presented in Table 9.2. Make a list of the ones that worked best for you and keep it as a handy reminder of what to do when urges to acquire or difficulty getting rid of items becomes a problem for you.

Dealing with Setbacks

If you experience setbacks in dealing with clutter, getting rid of items, and urges to acquire, there are various strategies you can use to get back on track. For example, you can call your clinician and set up an appointment if you need it, you can seek help from a friend or coach, and you can review your treatment notes. Remember to use cognitive strategies to avoid catastrophizing about the problem you have encountered. Also remember to use your problem-solving skills to deal with any problems you encounter, even serious ones.

Homework

- Review your *Workbook* and make a list of all the methods you've learned and highlight those you found most helpful.

- Review your Personal Session Forms to make a revised list of the ones that work best for you.

- Try out some skills you have not practiced for a while.

Conclusion

Congratulations! You are well on your way to overcoming your compulsive hoarding problem. With patience and continued effort, you will be able to maintain your progress and make even more gains.

Table 9.2 List of Treatment Techniques

Identify the methods below that worked best for you. Many of these apply not only to letting go of possessions, but also to resisting acquiring and to organizing.

- Review the Hoarding Model and consider the current state of affairs with regard to:
  - Personal and family vulnerabilities
  - Information processing problems
  - Thoughts and reasons for saving
  - Positive and negative emotions
  - Acquiring, saving, and avoidance behaviors
- Review the functional analysis of acquiring episodes.
- Repeat the clutter, unclutter, and ideal home visualizations to determine your reactions.
- Review your Personal Goals.
- If initial barriers to working on hoarding were identified, review progress on these.
- Acquiring—examine and review the following:
  - Acquiring Form to see progress and determine whether unwanted items continue to come into the home
  - Acquiring Questions Form
  - Your rules for acquiring
  - Hierarchy of acquiring situation to determine additional work needed
  - Progress on alternative sources of enjoyment
  - Faulty thinking about acquiring
  - Cognitive strategies—Downward Arrow, Need versus Want
- Review Problem-Solving Steps.
- Review strategies for keeping your attention focused.
- Review Personal Organizing Plan and Filing Paper Form:
  - Keep discarding decisions simple: trash, recycle, sell, donate.
  - Keep supplies on hand for organizing.
  - Review progress on "only handle it once" (OHIO) rule.
  - Implement decisions as soon as possible.
  - Review rules for how long to save paper.
  - Schedule times to organize and file.
  - Keep surfaces clear to prevent re-cluttering.
- Notice and correct problematic avoidance behaviors related to acquiring, sorting, and discarding.
- Review Questions About Possessions Form and/or Rules for Saving that facilitate decision-making.
- Review Thought Listing Exercise Form.
- Review Behavioral Experiment Form.
- Review imagined exposures to discarding and loss of possessions and information.
- Review the following cognitive strategies for parting with possessions:
  - Problematic Thinking Styles list
  - Questions About Possessions Form
  - Advantages/Disadvantages Worksheet
  - Downward Arrow
  - Examine the evidence for keeping or discarding items.
  - Thought Record Form
  - Need versus Want
  - Perfectionism Scale
  - Valuing Time
- Plan social activities outside your home.
- Invite others to visit you at home.
- Schedule self-treatment sessions.

Keep in mind that you have vulnerabilities that led to your hoarding in the first place. These emotional and behavioral habits are part of you, but like most people, you can overcome them so you have control over your behavior. Your best allies in the struggle against tendencies to acquire and save too many things are your new skills and your social supports, including your clinician and supportive family members and friends.

Appendices

1. Personal Session Form (chapter 2)

2. Instructions for Coaches (chapter 2)

3. Scoring Key for Assessments (chapters 2 & 9)

4. Brief Thought Record (chapter 3)

5. Hoarding Model (chapter 3)

6. Practice Form (chapter 4)

7. Downward Arrow Form (chapters 5 and 8)

8. Acquiring Questions Form (chapter 5)

9. Task List (chapter 6)

10. Personal Organizing Plan (chapter 6)

11. Preparing for Organizing Form (chapter 6)

12. Thought Listing Exercise Form (chapter 7)

13. Questions About Possessions Form (chapter 7)

14. Behavioral Experiment Form (chapter 7)

15. Thought Record Form (chapter 8)

All forms and worksheets in the Appendices are available for download and printing at www.oup.com/us/ttw

Personal Session Form

Initials: _____   Session #: _____   Date: _____

Agenda:

_____

_____

_____

Main Points:

_____

_____

_____

_____

_____

Homework:

_____

_____

_____

_____

_____

To Discuss Next Time:

_____

_____

_____

_____

_____

Personal Session Form

Initials: _____   Session #: _____   Date: _____

Agenda:

_____

_____

_____

Main Points:

_____

_____

_____

_____

_____

_____

Homework:

_____

_____

_____

_____

_____

_____

To Discuss Next Time:

_____

_____

_____

_____

_____

_____

Personal Session Form

Initials: _____   Session #: _____   Date: _____

Agenda:

_____

_____

_____

Main Points:

_____

_____

_____

_____

_____

_____

Homework:

_____

_____

_____

_____

_____

To Discuss Next Time:

_____

_____

_____

_____

_____

_____

Personal Session Form

Initials: _____   Session #: _____   Date: _____

Agenda:

_____

_____

_____

Main Points:

_____

_____

_____

_____

_____

_____

Homework:

_____

_____

_____

_____

_____

To Discuss Next Time:

_____

_____

_____

_____

_____

_____

Personal Session Form

Initials: _____   Session #: _____   Date: _____

Agenda:

_____

_____

_____

Main Points:

_____

_____

_____

_____

_____

_____

Homework:

_____

_____

_____

_____

_____

_____

To Discuss Next Time:

_____

_____

_____

_____

_____

_____

Personal Session Form

Initials: _____   Session #: _____   Date: _____

Agenda:

_____

_____

_____

Main Points:

_____

_____

_____

_____

_____

_____

Homework:

_____

_____

_____

_____

_____

_____

To Discuss Next Time:

_____

_____

_____

_____

_____

_____

Personal Session Form

Initials: _____   Session #: _____   Date: _____

Agenda:

_____

_____

_____

Main Points:

_____

_____

_____

_____

_____

_____

Homework:

_____

_____

_____

_____

_____

_____

To Discuss Next Time:

_____

_____

_____

_____

_____

_____

Personal Session Form

Initials: _____   Session #: _____   Date: _____

Agenda:

_____

_____

_____

Main Points:

_____

_____

_____

_____

_____

_____

Homework:

_____

_____

_____

_____

_____

_____

To Discuss Next Time:

_____

_____

_____

_____

_____

_____

Personal Session Form

Initials: _____   Session #: _____   Date: _____

Agenda:

_____

_____

_____

Main Points:

_____

_____

_____

_____

_____

_____

Homework:

_____

_____

_____

_____

_____

_____

To Discuss Next Time:

_____

_____

_____

_____

_____

_____

_____

Personal Session Form

Initials: _____   Session #: _____   Date: _____

Agenda:

_____

_____

_____

Main Points:

_____

_____

_____

_____

_____

_____

Homework:

_____

_____

_____

_____

_____

_____

To Discuss Next Time:

_____

_____

_____

_____

_____

_____

Personal Session Form

Initials: _____   Session #: _____   Date: _____

Agenda:

_____

_____

_____

Main Points:

_____

_____

_____

_____

_____

_____

_____

Homework:

_____

_____

_____

_____

_____

_____

To Discuss Next Time:

_____

_____

_____

_____

_____

_____

Personal Session Form

Initials: _____   Session #: _____   Date: _____

Agenda:

_____

_____

_____

Main Points:

_____

_____

_____

_____

_____

_____

Homework:

_____

_____

_____

_____

_____

_____

To Discuss Next Time:

_____

_____

_____

_____

_____

_____

Personal Session Form

Initials: _____   Session #: _____   Date: _____

Agenda:

_____

_____

_____

Main Points:

_____

_____

_____

_____

_____

_____

Homework:

_____

_____

_____

_____

_____

_____

To Discuss Next Time:

_____

_____

_____

_____

_____

_____

Personal Session Form

Initials: _____   Session #: _____   Date: _____

Agenda:

_____

_____

_____

Main Points:

_____

_____

_____

_____

_____

_____

Homework:

_____

_____

_____

_____

_____

_____

To Discuss Next Time:

_____

_____

_____

_____

_____

_____

Personal Session Form

Initials: _____   Session #: _____   Date: _____

Agenda:

_____

_____

_____

Main Points:

_____

_____

_____

_____

_____

_____

_____

Homework:

_____

_____

_____

_____

_____

_____

To Discuss Next Time:

_____

_____

_____

_____

_____

_____

Personal Session Form

Initials: _____   Session #: _____   Date: _____

Agenda:

_____

_____

_____

Main Points:

_____

_____

_____

_____

_____

_____

Homework:

_____

_____

_____

_____

_____

_____

To Discuss Next Time:

_____

_____

_____

_____

_____

_____

Personal Session Form

Initials: _____   Session #: _____   Date: _____

Agenda:

_____

_____

_____

Main Points:

_____

_____

_____

_____

_____

Homework:

_____

_____

_____

_____

_____

To Discuss Next Time:

_____

_____

_____

_____

_____

_____

Personal Session Form

Initials: _____   Session #: _____   Date: _____

Agenda:

_____

_____

_____

Main Points:

_____

_____

_____

_____

_____

_____

_____

Homework:

_____

_____

_____

_____

_____

To Discuss Next Time:

_____

_____

_____

_____

_____

_____

Personal Session Form

Initials: _____   Session #: _____   Date: _____

Agenda:

_____

_____

_____

Main Points:

_____

_____

_____

_____

_____

_____

Homework:

_____

_____

_____

_____

_____

To Discuss Next Time:

_____

_____

_____

_____

_____

_____

Personal Session Form

Initials: _____   Session #: _____   Date: _____

Agenda:

_____

_____

_____

Main Points:

_____

_____

_____

_____

_____

_____

Homework:

_____

_____

_____

_____

_____

_____

To Discuss Next Time:

_____

_____

_____

_____

_____

_____

Instructions for Coaches

Overcoming compulsive hoarding is often very difficult. Many people find it extremely helpful to have a support person or "coach" who can assist them with the process. As a coach, you will work together as a team with the clinician and the person with the hoarding problem. This guide outlines some ways to make your involvement most helpful.

Compulsive hoarding is not a single, simple problem, but consists of several interconnected problems. These usually include:

- *Excessive clutter*: This is the most easily recognized symptom of hoarding. Often, the clutter becomes so overwhelming that the person has a hard time knowing where to start.

- *Problems organizing and making decisions*: People with hoarding problems may have difficulty thinking clearly about their clutter or what to do about it. They may have a hard time recognizing the difference between items that are useful versus non-useful, valuable versus non-valuable, or sentimental versus non-sentimental. Therefore, to be on the safe side, they may treat all items as if they are useful, valuable, or sentimental. This leads to difficulty deciding when it is time to throw something out.

- *Difficulty letting go of possessions*: One of the most striking problems is difficulty letting go of and removing things—discarding, recycling, selling, and giving away items. This occurs even with items that seem to have little or no value. The amount of distress associated with removing clutter is often enormous.

- *A tendency to avoid or procrastinate*: People with hoarding problems often feel very overwhelmed by the sheer volume of clutter and the difficult task of decision-making. They may also feel depressed or nervous, which can add to a sense of fatigue and a tendency to avoid taking action. As a result, the person with hoarding is often tempted to decide, "This is too big to tackle today. I'll do it tomorrow."

- *Difficulty resisting urges to acquire objects*: For many people with hoarding problems, the urge to acquire things can be very strong, almost irresistible. Some people may feel a need to buy things; others may feel a need to pick up free things.

Not everyone who hoards has all of these problems. Every person and every hoarding problem are a little bit different, but all involve strong emotional reactions to possessions, thoughts and beliefs about saving things that may not always seem rational to you, and behaviors that enable the problem to persist. As part of the treatment program, the clinician will carefully review these aspects of hoarding with the person you are assisting and determine which problems are particularly troublesome. This is important, because the particular kinds of problems the person is facing guide what interventions to use.

We recommend coaches do the following:

- *Meet as a team* with the clinician and the person with the hoarding problem. Three people working together is a recipe for success, whereas three people working in different directions is unlikely to work.

- *Help the person remain focused* on the task in front of them. People with hoarding problems often find themselves easily distracted, especially when they are trying to reduce clutter, make decisions about possessions, or resist the urge to acquire things. Often, the coach can be very helpful by politely reminding the person what they are supposed to be doing right now.

- *Provide emotional support.* Because people who hoard have often been criticized by others, it is very important not to act like a taskmaster as this just makes people feel nervous or angry and interferes with their ability to learn new approaches. Use a gentle touch and when it feels right to you, express sympathy with statements such as, "I can see how hard this is for you" or "I understand that you have mixed feelings about whether to tackle this clutter." The person with the hoarding problem is going through some major stress and often needs a sympathetic ear or even a shoulder to cry on.

- *Help the person make decisions but DO NOT make decisions for them.* During treatment, the person with the hoarding problem is learning to develop new rules for deciding what to keep and what to remove. The coach can remind the person of these rules by asking questions, but not by telling them what to do. Ask them to simply talk out loud about their decision-making process for saving and discarding an item. Your task is not to convince them to get rid of things, but just to support them while they work through the process of making a decision. It may seem tedious, but often your mere presence will speed them along.

- *Be a cheerleader.* Sometimes, we all need an extra boost when things get difficult. Calling the person to remind them of their homework assignment, telling them you believe they can do it, and noticing when they are doing a good job are all good cheerleading strategies. But at the same time, don't do too much of this or the encouragement will seem burdensome and the praise hollow.

- *Help with hauling.* Many people who hoard have accumulated so much clutter that it would take them a year or more to discard it all by themselves. This makes it easy to get discouraged because progress is slow. Coaches are very helpful when they roll up their sleeves and help remove items from the home, so long as the person with hoarding makes all the decisions and remains fully in charge of the process.

- *Accompany the person on non-acquiring trips.* For people who acquire too many things, treatment often requires going to tempting stores or yard sales and not buying anything. It can be extremely helpful to have someone go with them to help resist temptation and make the trip a success.

We have also found that even the most well-meaning coaches can make themselves less helpful by using the wrong strategies. Here are some DON'Ts:

- *Don't argue* with the person about what to get rid of and what to acquire. Long debates about the usefulness of an item or the need to get rid of it will only produce negative emotional reactions that don't facilitate progress. Instead, whenever you feel in conflict, take a break, relax a bit, and remind yourself how difficult this is for the person.

- *Don't take over decisions.* It would certainly be easier and quicker if coaches simply took charge, decided what should stay and what should go, and hauled the clutter out themselves. But this method doesn't teach people how to manage their problem. The clutter will just build up again. Instead, be sure the person with hoarding is in charge at all times and makes all decisions, with the coach's support and guidance.

- *Don't touch or move anything without permission.* Imagine how you would feel if a well-meaning person came into your home and handled your things without permission. Doing this can damage the trust between you and make it impossible for the person to proceed.

- *Don't tell the person how they should feel.* It can be very hard to understand why someone feels so sentimental about keeping what looks like trash to you or fearful about getting rid of something that is clearly useless. But these feelings developed for reasons even the client may not yet understand. Be as patient as you can. We know that coaching can be frustrating.

- *Don't work beyond your own tolerance level.* To be a good coach, you have to take care of yourself first and then help your friend or family member. So feel free to set limits on how long and how much work you can do on any given occasion. Pat yourself on the back for your own efforts; helping someone who hoards is very hard work.

We hope these guidelines are helpful in working with someone who has a hoarding problem.

Scoring Key for Assessments

Hoarding Rating Scale (HRS)

Total score = sum of all 5 items Range = 0–40

Saving Inventory–Revised (SI-R)

Clutter Subscale (Nine Items)

Sum items: 1, 3, 5, 8, 10, 12, 15, 20, 22

Difficulty Discarding/Saving Subscale (Seven Items)

Sum items: 4 (reverse score), 6, 7, 13, 17, 19, 23

Acquisition Subscale (Seven Items)

Sum items: 2 (reverse score), 9, 11, 14, 16, 18, 21

Total score = sum of all items

Range = 0–92

Saving Cognitions Inventory (SCI)

Emotional Attachment (10 items)

Sum items: 1, 3, 6, 8, 9, 10, 13, 16, 22, 23

Control (three items)

Sum items: 5, 18, 24

Responsibility (six items)

Sum items: 2, 7, 11, 12, 15, 19

Memory (five items)

Sum items: 4, 14, 17, 20, 21

Total score = sum of all items

Range = 0–168

Activities of Daily Living–Hoarding (ADL-H)

Total score = sum all 15 items after excluding those rated "Not Applicable"; divide the summed score by the number of items given a numerical rating. This will yield an average of all applicable items.

Range = 1–5

Safety Questions

Examine individual items rated 2 and above to identify problematic areas requiring immediate attention.

Home Environment Inventory (HEI)

Total score = sum all items

Range = 0–45

Items rated 2 or above may indicate continuing problems.

Brief Thought Record

Initials: _____   Date: _____

Trigger Situation	Thought or Belief	Emotions	Actions/Behaviors

Brief Thought Record

Initials: _____   Date: _____

Trigger Situation	Thought or Belief	Emotions	Actions/Behaviors

Brief Thought Record

Initials: _____   Date: _____

Trigger Situation	Thought or Belief	Emotions	Actions/Behaviors

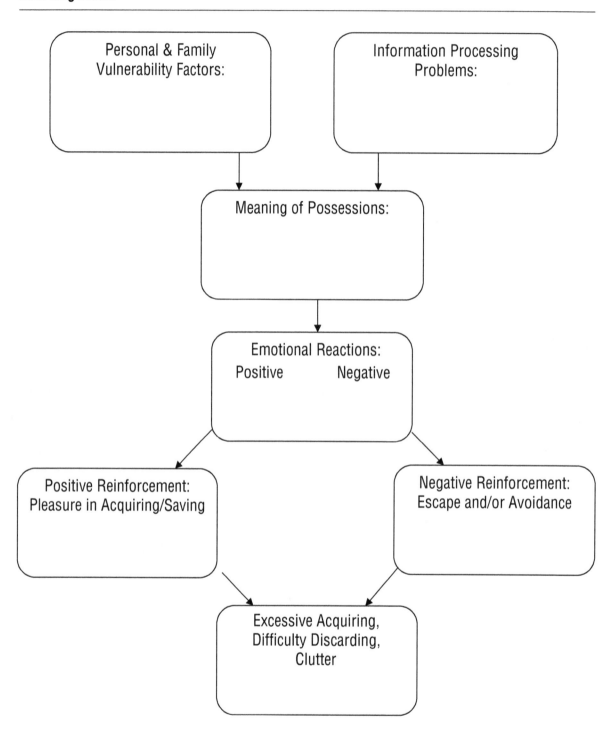

Practice Form

A. What was the item (to remove or not acquire)? _____

_____

Initial discomfort (0 = none to 100 = max)

_____

_____

B. What did you do (not acquire, trash, recycle, give away, other)? _____

_____

_____

_____

Discomfort rating (0 to 100)　　after 10 mins　　_____

after 20 mins　　_____

after 30 mins　　_____

after 40 mins　　_____

after 50 mins　　_____

after 1 hour　　_____

after next day　　_____

C. Conclusion regarding experiment: _____

_____

_____

_____

_____

_____

Practice Form

A. What was the item (to remove or not acquire)? _____

_____

Initial discomfort (0 = none to 100 = max)

_____

_____

B. What did you do (not acquire, trash, recycle, give away, other)? _____

_____

_____

_____

Discomfort rating (0 to 100)   after 10 mins _____

after 20 mins _____

after 30 mins _____

after 40 mins _____

after 50 mins _____

after 1 hour _____

after next day _____

C. Conclusion regarding experiment: _____

_____

_____

_____

_____

_____

_____

Practice Form

A. What was the item (to remove or not acquire)? _____

_____

   Initial discomfort (o = none to 100 = max)

_____

_____

B. What did you do (not acquire, trash, recycle, give away, other)? _____

_____

_____

_____

   Discomfort rating (o to 100)   after 10 mins   _____

                                    after 20 mins   _____

                                    after 30 mins   _____

                                    after 40 mins   _____

                                    after 50 mins   _____

                                    after 1 hour   _____

                                    after next day   _____

C. Conclusion regarding experiment: _____

_____

_____

_____

_____

_____

_____

Practice Form

A. What was the item (to remove or not acquire)? _____

_____

    Initial discomfort (0 = none to 100 = max)

_____

_____

B. What did you do (not acquire, trash, recycle, give away, other)? _____

_____

_____

_____

    Discomfort rating (0 to 100)   after 10 mins _____

                                     after 20 mins _____

                                     after 30 mins _____

                                     after 40 mins _____

                                     after 50 mins _____

                                     after 1 hour _____

                                     after next day _____

C. Conclusion regarding experiment: _____

_____

_____

_____

_____

_____

_____

Practice Form

A. What was the item (to remove or not acquire)? _____

_____

Initial discomfort (0 = none to 100 = max)

_____

_____

B. What did you do (not acquire, trash, recycle, give away, other)? _____

_____

_____

_____

Discomfort rating (0 to 100)   after 10 mins   _____

after 20 mins   _____

after 30 mins   _____

after 40 mins   _____

after 50 mins   _____

after 1 hour   _____

after next day   _____

C. Conclusion regarding experiment: _____

_____

_____

_____

_____

_____

_____

Practice Form

A. What was the item (to remove or not acquire)? _____

_____

Initial discomfort (0 = none to 100 = max)

_____

_____

B. What did you do (not acquire, trash, recycle, give away, other)? _____

_____

_____

_____

Discomfort rating (0 to 100)   after 10 mins   _____

after 20 mins   _____

after 30 mins   _____

after 40 mins   _____

after 50 mins   _____

after 1 hour   _____

after next day   _____

C. Conclusion regarding experiment: _____

_____

_____

_____

_____

_____

_____

Downward Arrow Form

Item: _____

In thinking about not acquiring or getting rid of (discarding, recycling, selling, giving away) this, what thoughts occur to you?

_____

_____

If you didn't acquire or got rid of this, what do you think would happen?

_____

_____

If this were true, why would it be so upsetting? (What would it mean to you? Why would that be so bad?)

_____

_____

If that were true, what's so bad about that?

_____

_____

What's the worst part about that?

_____

_____

What does that mean about *you?*

_____

_____

Downward Arrow Form

Item: _____

In thinking about not acquiring or getting rid of (discarding, recycling, selling, giving away) this, what thoughts occur to you?

_____

_____

If you didn't acquire or got rid of this, what do you think would happen?

_____

_____

If this were true, why would it be so upsetting? (What would it mean to you? Why would that be so bad?)

_____

_____

If that were true, what's so bad about that?

_____

_____

What's the worst part about that?

_____

_____

What does that mean about *you?*

_____

_____

Downward Arrow Form

Item: _____

In thinking about not acquiring or getting rid of (discarding, recycling, selling, giving away) this, what thoughts occur to you?

_____

_____

If you didn't acquire or got rid of this, what do you think would happen?

_____

_____

If this were true, why would it be so upsetting? (What would it mean to you? Why would that be so bad?)

_____

_____

If that were true, what's so bad about that?

_____

_____

What's the worst part about that?

_____

_____

What does that mean about *you?*

_____

_____

Acquiring Questions Form

- Does it fit with my own personal values?

- Do I have a real need for this item (not just a wish to have it)?

- Do I already own something similar?

- Am I only buying this because I feel bad (angry, depressed, etc.) right now?

- In a week, will I regret getting this?

- Could I manage without it?

- If it needs fixing, do I have enough time to do this or is my time better spent on other activities?

- Will I actually use this item in the near future?

- Do I have a specific place to put this?

- Is this truly valuable or useful or does it just seem so because I'm looking at it now?

- Is it good quality (accurate, reliable, attractive)?

- Will *not* getting this help me solve my hoarding problem?

_____

_____

_____

_____

_____

_____

_____

_____

_____

Task List

Priority Rating	Task	Date Put on List	Date Completed
A			
B			
C			

Task List

Priority Rating	Task	Date Put on List	Date Completed
A			
B			
C			

Task List

Priority Rating	Task	Date Put on List	Date Completed
A			
B			
C			

Task List

Priority Rating	Task	Date Put on List	Date Completed
A			
B			
C			

Task List

Priority Rating	Task	Date Put on List	Date Completed
A			
B			
C			

Personal Organizing Plan

Target area: _____

Item category	Final location
1. _____	_____
2. _____	_____
3. _____	_____
4. _____	_____
5. _____	_____
6. _____	_____
7. _____	_____
8. _____	_____
9. _____	_____
10. _____	_____
11. _____	_____
12. _____	_____
13. _____	_____
14. _____	_____
15. _____	_____
16. _____	_____
17. _____	_____
18. _____	_____
19. _____	_____
20. _____	_____

Personal Organizing Plan

Target area: _____

Item category	**Final location**
1. _____	_____
2. _____	_____
3. _____	_____
4. _____	_____
5. _____	_____
6. _____	_____
7. _____	_____
8. _____	_____
9. _____	_____
10. _____	_____
11. _____	_____
12. _____	_____
13. _____	_____
14. _____	_____
15. _____	_____
16. _____	_____
17. _____	_____
18. _____	_____
19. _____	_____
20. _____	_____

Personal Organizing Plan

Target area: _____

Item category	Final location
1. _____	_____
2. _____	_____
3. _____	_____
4. _____	_____
5. _____	_____
6. _____	_____
7. _____	_____
8. _____	_____
9. _____	_____
10. _____	_____
11. _____	_____
12. _____	_____
13. _____	_____
14. _____	_____
15. _____	_____
16. _____	_____
17. _____	_____
18. _____	_____
19. _____	_____
20. _____	_____

Preparing for Organizing Form

Room selection: _____

Target area or type of object selected: _____

Things I need to do to prepare for organizing:

1. _____

   _____

2. _____

   _____

3. _____

   _____

4. _____

   _____

5. _____

   _____

6. _____

   _____

Suggested tasks include:

- Getting boxes or storage containers

- Getting labels for boxes

- Clearing space for interim and final destinations

- Clearing space for sorting

- Scheduling times for working

Preparing for Organizing Form

Room selection: _____

Target area or type of object selected: _____

Things I need to do to prepare for organizing:

1. _____

   _____

2. _____

   _____

3. _____

   _____

4. _____

   _____

5. _____

   _____

6. _____

   _____

Suggested tasks include:

- Getting boxes or storage containers

- Getting labels for boxes

- Clearing space for interim and final destinations

- Clearing space for sorting

- Scheduling times for working

Preparing for Organizing Form

Room selection: _____

Target area or type of object selected: _____

Things I need to do to prepare for organizing:

1. _____

   _____

2. _____

   _____

3. _____

   _____

4. _____

   _____

5. _____

   _____

6. _____

   _____

Suggested tasks include:

- Getting boxes or storage containers

- Getting labels for boxes

- Clearing space for interim and final destinations

- Clearing space for sorting

- Scheduling times for working

Thought Listing Exercise Form

Initials _____ Date _____

Selected Item:

Anticipated Distress Rating (from 0=none to 100=maximum): _____

Predicted Duration of Distress: _____

Thoughts about Discarding: _____

Discarding Decision (circle): *Discard or Keep*

Distress rating after Decision: _____

Distress rating after 5 minutes: _____

Distress rating after 10 minutes: _____

Distress rating after 15 minutes: _____

Distress rating after 20 minutes: _____

Distress rating after 25 minutes: _____

Distress rating after 30 minutes: _____

Notes from Exercise:

_____

_____

_____

_____

_____

_____

_____

Thought Listing Exercise Form

Initials _____   Date _____

Selected Item:

Anticipated Distress Rating (from 0=none to 100=maximum): _____

Predicted Duration of Distress: _____

Thoughts about Discarding: _____

Discarding Decision (circle):   *Discard or Keep*

Distress rating after Decision: _____

Distress rating after 5 minutes: _____

Distress rating after 10 minutes: _____

Distress rating after 15 minutes: _____

Distress rating after 20 minutes: _____

Distress rating after 25 minutes: _____

Distress rating after 30 minutes: _____

Notes from Exercise:

_____

_____

_____

_____

_____

_____

_____

Thought Listing Exercise Form

Initials _____   Date _____

Selected Item:

Anticipated Distress Rating (from 0=none to 100=maximum): _____

Predicted Duration of Distress: _____

Thoughts about Discarding: _____

Discarding Decision (circle):   *Discard or Keep*

Distress rating after Decision: _____

Distress rating after 5 minutes: _____

Distress rating after 10 minutes: _____

Distress rating after 15 minutes: _____

Distress rating after 20 minutes: _____

Distress rating after 25 minutes: _____

Distress rating after 30 minutes: _____

Notes from Exercise:

_____

_____

_____

_____

_____

_____

_____

Thought Listing Exercise Form

Initials _____ Date _____

Selected Item:

Anticipated Distress Rating (from 0=none to 100=maximum): _____

Predicted Duration of Distress: _____

Thoughts about Discarding: _____

Discarding Decision (circle): *Discard or Keep*

Distress rating after Decision: _____

Distress rating after 5 minutes: _____

Distress rating after 10 minutes: _____

Distress rating after 15 minutes: _____

Distress rating after 20 minutes: _____

Distress rating after 25 minutes: _____

Distress rating after 30 minutes: _____

Notes from Exercise:

_____

_____

_____

_____

_____

_____

_____

Thought Listing Exercise Form

Initials _____ Date _____

Selected Item:

Anticipated Distress Rating (from 0=none to 100=maximum): _____

Predicted Duration of Distress: _____

Thoughts about Discarding: _____

Discarding Decision (circle):   *Discard or Keep*

Distress rating after Decision: _____

Distress rating after 5 minutes: _____

Distress rating after 10 minutes: _____

Distress rating after 15 minutes: _____

Distress rating after 20 minutes: _____

Distress rating after 25 minutes: _____

Distress rating after 30 minutes: _____

Notes from Exercise:

_____

_____

_____

_____

_____

_____

_____

Questions About Possessions Form

Sample Questions:

- How many do I already have and is that enough?

- Do I have enough time to use, review, or read it?

- Have I used this during the past year?

- Do I have a specific plan to use this item within a reasonable time frame?

- Does this fit with my own values and needs?

- How does this compare with the things I value highly?

- Does this just seem important because I'm looking at it now?

- Is it current?

- Is it of good quality, accurate, and/or reliable?

- Is it easy to understand?

- Would I buy it again if I didn't already own it?

- Do I really need it?

- Could I get it again if I found I really needed it?

- Do I have enough space for this?

- Will not having this help me solve my hoarding problem?

Questions About Possessions Form

- _____

- _____

- _____

- _____

- _____

- _____

- _____

- _____

- _____

- _____

- _____

Behavioral Experiment Form

Initials: _____ Date: _____

1. Behavioral experiment to be completed: _____

_____

_____

2. What do you predict (are afraid) will happen? _____

_____

_____

3. How strongly do you believe this will happen (0–100%) _____

_____

4. Initial discomfort (0–100) _____

5. What actually happened? _____

_____

_____

_____

_____

6. Final discomfort (0–100) _____

7. Did your predictions come true? _____

8. What conclusions do you draw from this experiment? _____

_____

_____

_____

_____

Behavioral Experiment Form

Initials: _____   Date: _____

1. Behavioral experiment to be completed: _____
   _____
   _____

2. What do you predict (are afraid) will happen? _____
   _____
   _____

3. How strongly do you believe this will happen (0–100%) _____
   _____

4. Initial discomfort (0–100) _____

5. What actually happened? _____
   _____
   _____
   _____
   _____

6. Final discomfort (0–100) _____

7. Did your predictions come true? _____

8. What conclusions do you draw from this experiment? _____
   _____
   _____
   _____
   _____

Behavioral Experiment Form

Initials: _____   Date: _____

1. Behavioral experiment to be completed: _____

    _____

    _____

2. What do you predict (are afraid) will happen? _____

    _____

    _____

3. How strongly do you believe this will happen (0–100%) _____

    _____

4. Initial discomfort (0–100) _____

5. What actually happened? _____

    _____

    _____

    _____

    _____

6. Final discomfort (0–100) _____

7. Did your predictions come true? _____

8. What conclusions do you draw from this experiment? _____

    _____

    _____

    _____

    _____

Behavioral Experiment Form

Initials: _____   Date: _____

1. Behavioral experiment to be completed: _____

    _____

    _____

2. What do you predict (are afraid) will happen? _____

    _____

    _____

3. How strongly do you believe this will happen (0–100%) _____

    _____

4. Initial discomfort (0–100) _____

5. What actually happened? _____

    _____

    _____

    _____

    _____

6. Final discomfort (0–100) _____

7. Did your predictions come true? _____

8. What conclusions do you draw from this experiment? _____

    _____

    _____

    _____

    _____

Behavioral Experiment Form

Initials: _____   Date: _____

1. Behavioral experiment to be completed: _____

    _____

    _____

2. What do you predict (are afraid) will happen? _____

    _____

    _____

3. How strongly do you believe this will happen (0–100%) _____

    _____

4. Initial discomfort (0–100) _____

5. What actually happened? _____

    _____

    _____

    _____

    _____

6. Final discomfort (0–100) _____

7. Did your predictions come true? _____

8. What conclusions do you draw from this experiment? _____

    _____

    _____

    _____

    _____

Thought Record Form

Initials: _____   Date: _____

Trigger situation	Thoughts	Emotions	Rational alternative	Outcome

Thought Record Form

Initials: _____   Date: _____

Trigger situation	Thoughts	Emotions	Rational alternative	Outcome

Thought Record Form

Initials: _____ Date: _____

Trigger situation	Thoughts	Emotions	Rational alternative	Outcome

Thought Record Form

Initials: _____   Date: _____

Trigger situation	Thoughts	Emotions	Rational alternative	Outcome

Thought Record Form

Initials: _____ Date: _____

Trigger situation	Thoughts	Emotions	Rational alternative	Outcome

About the Authors

Gail Steketee, PhD, is Dean and Professor of the Boston University School of Social Work. She received her MSS and PhD from Bryn Mawr's Graduate School of Social Work and Social Research. Her research has focused on understanding the causes and consequences of obsessive-compulsive spectrum conditions, especially hoarding disorder, and on developing and testing evidence-based treatments for these conditions. She has received several grants from NIMH and from the International Obsessive Compulsive Disorder Foundation (IOCDF) to examine family factors that influence treatment outcomes for anxiety disorders and to test cognitive and behavioral treatments for OCD, hoarding disorder, and body dysmorphic disorder. Her research on hoarding with collaborators Drs. Randy Frost and David Tolin has contributed significantly to the development of diagnostic criteria for hoarding disorder in the major revision of the *Diagnostic and Statistical Manual for Mental Disorders* (DSM-5, 2013). Dr. Steketee has published over 200 articles and chapters and more than a dozen books on research findings and evidence-based treatments for OCD, hoarding, and related disorders. Her best-selling book *Stuff: Compulsive Hoarding and the Meaning of Things* (Houghton Mifflin Harcourt, 2010), co-authored with Dr. Frost, was a finalist for the Books for a Better Life Award. She is a Fellow in the American Academy of Social Work and Social Welfare and has received awards from the Association of Behavioral and Cognitive Therapies, the Society of Social Work Research, and the Aaron T. Beck Institute for Cognitive Studies. She serves on editorial boards and as ad hoc reviewer for multiple journals in social work, psychology, and psychiatry. She also serves on scientific advisory boards of U.S. and Canadian OCD foundations and on a Commission for the Council of Social Work Education. She has appeared in a variety of media venues regarding her work on hoarding.

Dr. Randy O. Frost is currently the Harold and Elsa Siipola Israel Professor of Psychology at Smith College. He received his PhD from the University of Kansas in 1977 following a doctoral internship at the University of Washington School of Medicine. He is an internationally recognized expert on obsessive-compulsive disorder and hoarding disorder and has published more than 150 scientific articles and book chapters on these topics. Dr. Frost serves on the Scientific Advisory Board of the International OCD Foundation and, with Dr. Gail Steketee, co-edits the Hoarding Center on the IOCDF website. He has co-authored several books on hoarding, including *Buried in Treasures: Help for Compulsive Acquiring, Saving, and Hoarding* (with Drs. David Tolin and Gail Steketee and published by Oxford University Press). *Buried in Treasures* received a Self-Help Book of Merit Award from the Association for Behavioral and Cognitive Therapy in 2010. His best-selling book, *Stuff: Compulsive Hoarding and the Meaning of Things* (with Gail Steketee), was published by Houghton Mifflin Harcourt in 2010 and was a finalist for the 2010 Books for a Better Life Award. *Stuff* was also named a Must Read Book for 2011 by Massachusetts Book Awards and has been translated into four languages. His work has been funded by the International Obsessive Compulsive Foundation and the National Institute of Mental Health. Dr. Frost is one of the original members of the Hoarding of Animals Research Consortium and has served as consultant to numerous communities in setting up task forces to deal with the problem of hoarding. In 2012 he was awarded the Lifetime Achievement Award for excellence in innovation, treatment, and research in the field of hoarding and cluttering by the Mental Health Association of San Francisco.

Index

Page numbers followed by "*f*" indicate a figure.

CPSIA information can be obtained
at www.ICGtesting.com
Printed in the USA
BVHW060228130422
633716BV00002B/10

9 780199 334940